'This book is a must-read for any professional or academic interested in psychology, Muslim or non-Muslim. Prof. Bagus Riyono is offering in its original contributions to the science of psychology, and making a case that the Islamic worldview is a natural foundation for human wellbeing, happiness and resilience.'

Jasser Auda, *PhD, professor, president of Maqasid Institute Global*

Tazkiya Therapy in Islāmic Psychotherapy

This book explores tazkiya therapy, a holistic psychological approach based on Qur'ânic guidance and rooted in the understanding of human beings as multidimensional – that is, physical, psychological, social and spiritual beings.

The book starts with a detailed explanation or the object, the process and the purpose of tazkiya therapy, along with an account of the boundaries and the enabling factors of the approach. Rather than a singular theoretical framework, tazkiya therapy is a dynamic and flexible approach that integrates multiple frameworks and disciplines to grow the human soul, cognition, emotion and behaviour. Although it is a multidimensional approach, the process of therapy is step-by-step, and the middle part of the book presents the key stages in the approach. Within these steps, the therapist is given seven different approaches that they can customise to the needs of the client depending on whether they need assistance with thinking patterns, emotional disturbance, a behavioural problem or a dysfunctional nervous system. The book ends with a comprehensive summary of the model, a series of case studies, a future outlook on training and an application for continuing the study and practice of tazkiya therapy.

This book, based on the foundation that tazkiya therapy covers issues that are spiritual in nature and always connects to Allâh in facilitating the healing process, will fulfil the needs of practicing Muslim psychologists, psychiatrists and students of psychology and Islāmic studies.

Dr Bagus Riyono, MA, is currently the president of the International Association of Muslim Psychologists (IAMP). He is also a faculty member of the psychology department of Gadjah Mada University, Indonesia, and head of the Islāmic Psychology Study Group. Currently, he is working on the application of his theories in a cognitive–spiritual intervention called tazkiya therapy.

Focus Series on Islāmic Psychology

Series Editor: Professor Dr. G. Hussein Rassool, Professor of Islāmic Psychology.

About the Series

In contemporary times, there is increasing focus on the need to adapt approaches of psychology, counselling psychology and psychotherapy to accommodate the integration of spirituality and psychology. With the increasing focus on the need to meet the wholistic needs of Muslims, there was a call to adapt approaches to the understanding of behaviour and experiences from an Islāmic epistemological and ontological worldview.

The aim of the Focus Series on Islāmic psychology and psychotherapy is to introduce a range of educational, clinical and research interventions relating to Islāmic psychology and psychotherapy that are authentic, practical, concise and based on cutting-edge research. Each volume focuses on a particular aspect of Islāmic psychology and psychotherapy, its application with a specific client group, a particular methodology or approach, or a critical analysis of existing and emergent theoretical and historical ideas.

Each book in the Focus Series is written, in accessible language, with the assumption that the readers have no prior knowledge of Islāmic psychology and psychotherapy.

Integrating Acceptance and Commitment Therapy with Islāmic Psychotherapy for Managing Chronic Pain (2024)
By Razia Bhatti-Ali

Integrating Spiritual Interventions in Islāmic Psychology: A Practical Guide (2024)
By Juraida Latif, Shaakirah Dockrat Boda, & G. Hussein Rassool

Islāmically Modified Cognitive Behavioural Therapy (2025)
By Mahdi Qasqas

Tazkiya Therapy in Islāmic Psychotherapy (2025)
Bagus Riyono

Tazkiya Therapy in Islāmic Psychotherapy

Bagus Riyono

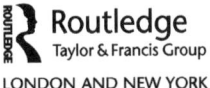

Routledge
Taylor & Francis Group

LONDON AND NEW YORK

First published 2025
by Routledge
4 Park Square, Milton Park, Abingdon, Oxon OX14 4RN

and by Routledge
605 Third Avenue, New York, NY 10158

Routledge is an imprint of the Taylor & Francis Group, an informa business

© 2025 Bagus Riyono

British Library Cataloguing-in-Publication Data
A catalogue record for this book is available from the British Library

Library of Congress Cataloging-in-Publication Data
Names: Riyono, Bagus, 1963– author.
Title: Tazkiya therapy in Islāmic psychotherapy / Bagus Riyono.
Other titles: Focus series on Islāmic psychology and psychotherapy
Description: Abingdon, Oxon : New York, NY : Routledge, 2025. | Series:
   Focus series on Islāmic psychology and psychotherapy | Includes
   bibliographical references and index.
Identifiers: LCCN 2024012871 (print) | LCCN 2024012872 (ebook) | ISBN
   9781032714691 (hardback) | ISBN 9781032717333 (paperback) | ISBN
   9781032717340 (ebook)
Subjects: MESH: Psychotherapy—methods | Islam | Religion and Psychology |
   Psychological Well-Being | Holistic Health | Case Reports
Classification: LCC RC480.5 (print) | LCC RC480.5 (ebook) | NLM WM 427 |
   DDC 616.89/14—dc23/eng/20240408
LC record available at https://lccn.loc.gov/2024012871
LC ebook record available at https://lccn.loc.gov/2024012872

ISBN: 9781032714691 (hbk)
ISBN: 9781032717333 (pbk)
ISBN: 9781032717340 (ebk)

DOI: 10.4324/9781032717340

Typeset in Times New Roman
by Apex CoVantage, LLC

Contents

Preface

Alhamdulillah, finally, this book on tazkiya therapy has been published. The process of writing this book began in 2011 when the author just finished his PhD at Universitas Gadjah Mada, Indonesia. In his PhD dissertation, he constructed three theories of human motivation and personality through a meta-ethnographic study. In the beginning, the author found that motivation is actually the core of psychological dynamics in every context. Motivation is the fundamental dynamics in working conditions, schools and education, and also psychotherapy. In general, conventional psychology focuses on human behaviour and tries to explain "why" and "how" certain behaviours take place. From this perspective, actually what is done in psychotherapy is to motivate the client to practise healthy behaviour to achieve mental health.

In 2016, the author encountered a new methodology to understand human beings as multidimensional beings from an Islāmic perspective. This methodology is called the Maqasid methodology. The author then studied the human soul from the Qur'ânic messages and found that the human soul is the essence of human beings. When an individual has a problem with their mental health, the root cause is found to be in the dynamics of the human soul. After studying deeper about the dynamics of the human soul, the author found very strong messages in the Qur'ân that the discipline to manage and develop the human soul is called tazkiya. Then the author started to develop the concept and application of tazkiya to achieve psychological health. This approach is called tazkiya therapy.

Along with the development of this book, the author started to apply the tazkiya therapy in several counselling sessions. The integration of the motivational theories, the Qur'ânic studies of the soul and the practical experience of practising tazkiya therapy are then compiled into this book.

This book is an initial effort to introduce tazkiya therapy as an alternative in psychotherapy that is based on the Qur'ânic messages, integrated with the scientific findings. This initial effort in applying the Islāmic paradigm to psychotherapy is needed since interest in Islāmic psychology is growing worldwide. We hope this book can contribute to the establishment of psychological science based on the Islāmic perspective. This book is aimed especially at Muslim psychologists and students around the world, but it is also open for other groups of readers who are interested in Islāmic thoughts and interventions.

This book will fulfil the needs of Muslim psychologists and psychiatrists and also students of psychology and psychiatry, mostly in Muslim countries and also for Muslim students around the world. The interest in Islāmic psychology is fast growing, and there are thousands of members of several professional associations on Islāmic psychology around the world. There are also accredited study programmes on psychology in several countries that adopt the Islāmic psychology approach, for example Charles Sturt University in Sydney, Australia; Universitas Muhammadiyah Surakarta, Indonesia; Riphah Institute in Pakistan; Cambridge Muslim College in England; International Islāmic University Malaysia in Malaysia; and more are in the process of establishment.

Acknowledgements

This book is a product of collaborative effort of many individuals who have contributed in various ways to make this book available. First of all, I would like to express my gratitude to Prof. Dr G. Hussein Rassool, who had motivated the author to write this book, also for Prof. Jasser Auda for inspiring the author on Maqasid Methodology. I am so grateful that I have learned a lot from Dr. Aly Abdel Moneim about the Maqasid Methodology. I am also thankful to Prof. Rasjid Skinner who has inspired me that it is possible to develop psychotherapy from an Islāmic perspective. I would like to also express my thanks to all my colleagues in the Faculty of Psychology of Universitas Gadjah Mada who have supported me in many ways.

This book would not be possible without the help of my six hardworking assistants, Alifah N. Istiqomah, Annisa A. Ayuningtyas, Hastinia Apriasari, Lulu'ul Jannah, Nur R. Itsnaini and Rahma A. Fachrunisa, who have worked days and nights to make sure this book can be finished on time. Last but not least, I really appreciate the support of my wife, Emi Zulaifah, who has been patient and supportive of my work, and also of all my children, Atika, Astari, Maghfira, Thoriq and Nafis, and my granddaughter, Lila, who have made me feel complete as a father and a grandpa.

About the Author

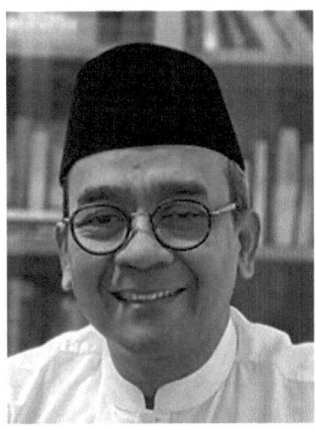

Dr Bagus Riyono, MA, is a senior lecturer of psychology in the Faculty of Psychology, Universitas Gadjah Mada, Indonesia. His expertise is in Islāmic psychology and industrial/organisational psychology. As an expert in Islāmic psychology, he also serves as the president of the International Association of Muslim Psychologists (IAMP), which is an international organisation for Muslim psychologists around the world.

Dr Riyono pursued his master's degree at Hofstra University (US) and his doctoral degree at Universitas Gadjah Mada (Indonesia). His doctoral dissertation about the theory of motivation has become a well-known theory in psychology globally. Overall, his research areas are about motivation, personality, leadership and organisational development.

Dr Riyono's research is focused on building a meta-theory in the field of human motivation that integrates all theories of motivation to become one

Grand Theory of human behaviour based on the worldview of Islam. He developed some theories on motivation and personality, including theory of anchor, theory of human motivation model, theory of R.U.H and theory of the layers of human soul. Recently, he is also conducting research on the theory of human potential. All of his research about human motivation and personality represents his great dedication towards the development of Islāmic psychology.

As a Muslim scholar, Dr Riyono has been a visiting lecturer and international speaker presenting his theories globally, such as in Charles Sturt University (Australia), Riphah International University (Pakistan), Moscow State University of Psychology and Education (Russia), Tatarstan Academy of Science (Russia), Universitat Leipzig (Germany), Rijksuniversiteit Groningen (Netherland) and J.F. Oberlin University (Japan). He also teaches in Avicenna Academy, a school of Islāmic psychology that provides education and research in Islāmic psychology based on the Qur'ân using the Maqasid method. In Universitas Gadjah Mada, he is the founder of the Islāmic psychology community, which is a group of lecturers and students who have interest in studying Islāmic psychology. Besides that, he also frequently teaches various courses on Islāmic psychology in Indonesian society and globally.

Dr Riyono has published numerous articles and books. His current work is about developing *tazkiya* therapy as a conceptual and practical guidance in promoting mental health and overcoming psychological problems. He is also developing a guidebook about the basics of psychology based on Islāmic psychology. To sum up, he is an internationally recognised Muslim scholar in psychology, teacher, researcher and author. Please visit www.bagusriyono. com for more information.

1 Introduction

This book is about an approach in psychotherapy that is based on Qur'ânic teachings. The keywords of Islāmic psychotherapy are *tazkiya* or "تزكية." *Tazkiya* means purification, nurturing, and growing. This book also argues that knowledge is the fundamental aspect of healing. Therefore, this book introduces seven theoretical frameworks as a multidimensional concept of psychological well-being and growth.

Tazkiya therapy is an approach for holistic psychological health based on Qur'ânic guidance. Tazkiya therapy is unique because it is a multidimensional, philosophically sound and theoretically rich approach. Tazkiya therapy is based on the understanding of human beings as a multidimensional being, that is physical, psychological, social and spiritual. This multidimensionality perspective of human beings is based on the Qur'ânic philosophy that illustrates human beings with multiple terminologies, for example *nafs, qalb, bašyar, insān, bani ādam, khalifah* and *abdullah*. Philosophically, human beings are created by Alláh with the purpose to go through a challenging life in this world in order to grow and to become worthy to meet Alláh in the Hereafter. Tazkiya therapy is also a theoretically rich approach, meaning it integrates any theoretical framework that is coherent with a philosophical perspective of human beings according to Al Qur'ân. For example, tazkiya therapy recognises and integrates theories about ego defence mechanism (Freud, 1961), human potential (Riyono, 2023), freedom and responsibility (Barrett, 2017), reinforcement (Skinner, 1971), self-actualisation (Maslow, 1970), meaning (Frankl, 1962), self-regulation (Deci et al., 1996) and anchor personality (Riyono, 2012). These theories are integrated in a system of understanding the multidimensional human beings and their psychological problems, as well as the appropriate therapeutic approach. In other words, tazkiya therapy is not an approach using a singular theoretical framework. Even though tazkiya therapy integrates multiple theoretical frameworks, it does not mean that it is a complicated approach; rather, it is a dynamic and flexible approach to grow the human soul, cognition, emotion, and behaviour.

Tazkiya therapy expands the concept of psychological health into a wider perspective of human well-being and uses the term psychological health

DOI: 10.4324/9781032717340-1

instead of mental health. Psychological health includes mental health but integrates with the treatment of the psyche, which is the human soul. By definition, mental health only deals with the mind, which is mostly cognitive in nature. Tazkiya therapy perceives human beings to have more potential beyond cognitive abilities, that is emotional and spiritual. Therefore, psychological health covers mental health, emotional health and spiritual health. However, tazkiya therapy uses the cognitive approach as a starting point because cognition is the entrance that can influence emotional and also spiritual health. In other words, the ideal condition of psychological health includes cognition, emotion and spirituality in a multidimensional fashion, but the process of therapy is through developing an understanding of the issues.

Since it is an Islāmic approach, tazkiya therapy is strongly attached with the belief and trust in Allāh the Almighty and the Most Knowing. However, it is also workable for clients who have not believed in Allāh yet. Tazkiya therapy is based on the worldview that all human beings are Allāh's creatures who will live forever beyond this worldly life. This worldview believes that all human beings are in the process of learning and developing towards the psychological state of a believer who surrenders to Allāh's will. Those who do not believe in Allāh are perceived as still in the middle of a journey and still in the process of learning. On the other hand, since life in this world is dynamic, those who already believe in Allāh are also facing the risk of forgetfulness. Tazkiya therapy, in this case, is an intervention to remind them to go back to the truth, or in Arabic *tawbah*, which means repentance.

The purpose of tazkiya therapy is not limited to happiness in this worldly life, but it stretches towards the eternity, which is the life in the Hereafter. This is fundamental as a mindset that will be endorsed throughout the process of tazkiya therapy. The orientation towards eternal life is essential since what we are focusing on in tazkiya therapy is the human soul. Since our focus is the human soul, life in this world is only temporary and very short. However, this worldly life will determine our happiness in the Hereafter. So, our worldly life is a journey, and the destination is our eternal life. The orientation towards the life in the Hereafter will also influence the happiness in the life in this world because it will strengthen our resilience, optimism, hope and patience in facing any problems.

In order to be able to do tazkiya, we need to develop knowledge from the signs that are revealed by Allāh through the Qur'ânic verses, the universe (natural science) and the dynamic of our souls (psychology and social science), as mentioned in Al-Qur'ân Surah Fussilat (41):53. The role of the therapist in tazkiya therapy is to facilitate the client's understanding of these signs through reason, empathy and spirituality. When the client succeeds in developing the knowledge through the process of tazkiya, they will obtain wisdom (*ḥikmah*) (Al-Baqarah (2):151; An-Nisā' (3):162; Al-Jumuah (62):2). When they become wiser, their soul grows to a higher level, as mentioned in Qur'ân Al-Mujadilah (58):11. The outcome of tazkiya therapy is *falāḥ*, which means to be successful through appropriate effort. The success that is promised by the process of tazkiya will require effort, so along the way, the individual (client) will develop knowledge and skills. The knowledge that is developed in the process of tazkiya therapy concerns the understanding of the essential human potential and characteristics, the understanding of the purpose of human life and the understanding of the dynamic of human life in this world: for example, the meaning of suffering; the nature of life uncertainty; and knowledge about essential values such as *šyukr* (gratitude), *ṣabr* (patience) and *istiqomah* (perseverance). Along with the acquisition of this knowledge, the client also develops skills to reframe and reinterpret their psychological problems, which will give them ideas on how to cope with these problems and how to solve them. By developing skills to deal with their own problems, the clients will be able to secure a sustainable success. This means that clients will be able to solve their own future problems because they have already acquired the skills. This explains why tazkiya therapy will minimise relapse because they will become independent and grow.

To understand deeper about the three sources of knowledge, that is the universe, the human soul and the Qur'ânic messages, we have to comprehend the meaning of those sources. The universe is the natural world that is material in nature and has certain characteristics that are observable. On the other hand, the human soul is an unseen reality that has different characteristics and different dynamics. The third source is the Al-Qur'ân, which is a narrated source of knowledge. The Qur'ânic messages cover both the observable realities and the unseen realities in an integrated manner.

The human soul is the focus of tazkiya therapy, so one needs a proper perspective to understand it and its dynamic. As an unseen reality, human souls cannot be treated as something that is material in nature. There are at least three fundamental differences between the human soul and the material realities. Firstly, materials are divisible into parts; for example, the human body is the part of the universe consisting of several parts, like the head, the hand, the legs and so on. On the other hand, the human soul reflects the human self, which includes the human mind that is not divisible. This relates to the term individual as the other representation of the self or the soul. The individual is indivisible. It is the other term that can substitute the self and the soul (Qur'ân An-Nisā' (4):1): "Allâh created human beings from one individual." The term individual in the translation refers to the Qur'ânic word *nafs*.

The second difference between observable realities and unseen realities is that unseen realities, the human soul, are not contained in time and space, whereas material reality is limited by time and space. That is why, the term here and now in psychology is not quite compatible when we talk about the human soul. This is evidenced in the case of imagination and memory that are the property of the human soul and are not contained in time and space. This is also evidenced in the phenomenon of dream.

The third difference between observable realities and the soul is that the soul has a multidimensional dynamic that can simultaneously happen. This reality has to be understood by a tazkiya therapist so that the process of tazkiya therapy follows these dynamics. It also means that the soul has the freedom to change anytime so that the tazkiya therapist's role is not to control these dynamics but rather to give directions and tolerate them.

The fourth difference between material reality and the unseen reality is that there is no such thing as increasing and decreasing the volume of the soul. The soul that is also called the heart is not changing in volume, but it can change in terms of direction, energy and attitude. This means that the human spiritual heart cannot be reduced or handicapped in any way, but it can be misguided, opened or closed, and purified or not purified. This reality is an advantage because the opportunity to be guided is always open, but sometimes the opportunity is not taken because of the attitude of the heart itself. In other words, no matter how big the problem of the heart is, it can always be solved. In religious terms, no matter how big the sin the heart has done, the opportunity to repentance is always open. So, this reality is very important for tazkiya therapists, so there is no need to give up no matter how difficult the psychological problem is.

The dynamic of these two realities cannot escape from Alláh's ruling. Everything that happens in the material world happens due to Alláh's will or Alláh's command. It is said in the Qur'ân that even any dry leaf that falls from the tree is in accordance with Alláh's plan (QS Al-An'am (06):56). The swinging of the spiritual heart is also in Alláh's hand. Nobody can change anybody's heart without Alláh's permission (Al-Baqarah (02):272; Yunus (10):99–100 and Al-Ghasyiyah (88):21–22). The unique characteristic of the spiritual heart that also differentiates from the material reality is that the heart has an independent will, and Alláh will not change anybody's heart if they do not have the will to do it (QS Ar-Ra'd (13):11). These realities are written in the Qur'ân as the word from Alláh. These also explained that the Qur'ân contained both realities, the universe, which is material in nature, and the reality of the human soul, which is immaterial or unseen.

The general protocol of tazkiya therapy is as follows:

a. The therapist listens empathetically to the clients' problems, emotionally and rationally.
b. The therapist explores further the possible causes of the clients' problems by digging into the past experience, emotional dynamics and rational understanding of these experiences.
c. The therapist leads the clients to confirm the core problem that they experienced, which might involve logical fallacy, extreme emotional arousal or limited perspective of the meaning of life.

d. If the clients are intelligent enough and open minded, they might be able to solve their problems independently after going through step 3. However, the therapist can offer support that can help the clients solve their problems.

e. In order to support the clients, the therapist decides where to start by using one of the seven approaches that is available and customises it with the needs of the clients. These seven approaches will be explained in Chapter 5 of this book.

f. Once the therapist finds the appropriate approach to the problem of the clients, he then goes deeper through the approach to help the clients solve the core of the problem.

g. The therapist directs the clients' thoughts, emotions and conscience towards the ideal state based on the selected approaches.

Before these protocols are applied, the tazkiya therapist should start with a prayer to Alláh to ask for Alláh's guidance in the process of therapy. This is important as well. Besides that, the therapist should ask the client to do a prayer also so that the clients are ready and open their heart for Alláh's guidance. It has to be understood that Alláh is always present along the process of tazkiya therapy, and both the therapist and the client should be ready for Alláh's decision. If the client does not believe in Alláh yet, at least the therapist could make sure that the client is willing to go through the process of the therapy sincerely and is ready to learn about themselves and the psychological problems. This initial step is the elaboration of what is called as *niyyah*, which means a conscious intention.

These protocols of tazkiya therapy can be called empathetic directives. The empathetic part is similar to other kinds of psychotherapy, but tazkiya therapy does not stop there. Since tazkiya therapy is based on Qur'ânic guidance, the treatment is continued to direct the client to the ideal psychological state based on the Qur'ânic teachings.

The application of tazkiya therapy is limited to psychological problems such as thinking pattern, emotional disturbance and behavioural disorder. Tazkiya therapy needs to be combined with an additional approach in dealing with mental problems that are caused by the dysfunctional nervous system.

Tazkiya therapy is an approach to psychological health, especially for Muslim psychologists or any psychologist who believes in God and the Hereafter. However, tazkiya therapy can be customised to be applied to anyone considering the individual differences.

This book contains chapters that explain the foundation of tazkiya therapy and the approach that can be used in tazkiya therapy. Chapter 2 reveals the seven realities of life based on a comprehensive study from Qur'ânic messages and the state of the art of psychological science. These seven realities of life provide the ground for tazkiya therapy that cannot be denied. Accepting these seven realities is a halfway to reach psychological health. These seven realities are the starting point in the process of tazkiya therapy that provides the baseline mindset.

Chapter 3 formulates the seven indicators of psychological health as the objective of tazkiya therapy. These seven indicators of psychological health are formulated based on Qur'ânic messages and the state-of-the-art of psychological science. These seven indicators are integrated in nature, and each of these indicators has influenced each other.

Chapter 4 describes the seven principles of tazkiya therapy that are based on Qur'ânic messages. These seven principles provide the foundation or the basic paradigms in tazkiya therapy that differentiate tazkiya therapy from other approaches in conventional psychology.

Chapter 5 elaborates the seven approaches of tazkiya therapy that respond to the seven realities of life and aim at the seven indicators of psychological health. These seven approaches also serve as the protocols of tazkiya therapy and are also integrated in nature. These seven approaches are not seven separate methods but seven entry points that will relate to each other and enrich each other. These seven approaches are not sequential in nature, but they should be applied and customised based on the issues and also the circumstances.

Chapter 6 illustrates tazkiya therapy in action by presenting several cases and the analysis of it. These cases are some examples to illustrate tazkiya therapy in action.

This book is aimed at providing the reader with the initial guidance of tazkiya therapy. Those who want to practise tazkiya therapy might need additional training based on this book to acquire this skill in practice. The content of this book provides the knowledge that is needed and has to be learned before the practice of tazkiya therapy. Those who want to practise tazkiya therapy also suggested expanding the knowledge by studying more deeply the Qur'ânic messages that are relevant to the issue of psychological health. The basic skills in counselling and psychotherapy also need to be developed through separate training programmes.

References

Barrett, L. F. (2017). *How emotions are made: The secret life of the brain.* Houghton Mifflin Harcourt.

Deci, E. L., Ryan, R. M., & Williams, G. C. (1996). Need satisfaction and the self-regulation of learning. *Learning and Individual Differences*, *8*(3), 165–183. https://doi.org/10.1016/S1041-6080(96)90013-8

Frankl, V. (1962). *Man's search for meaning* (English trans. I. Lasch). Beacon Press.

Freud, S. (1961). *Beyond the pleasure principle.* W.W. Norton and Company.

Maslow, A. H. (1970). *Motivation and personality* (2nd ed.). Harper and Row.

Riyono, B. (2023). Constructing the theory of human basic potential based on Qur'ânic messages: Study with Maqasid methodology. *Minbar Islāmic Studies*, *16*(2), 449–475. https://doi.org/10.31162/2618-9569-2023-16-2-449-475

Riyono, B., & Himam, F. (2012). In search for anchors the fundamental motivational force in compensating for human vulnerability. *Gadjah Mada International Journal of Business*, *14*(3), 229–252. https://doi.org/10.22146/gamaijib.5475

Skinner, B. F. (1971). *Beyond freedom and dignity*. Knopf/Random House.

2 The realities and the dynamics of human life

This chapter will explore the seven realities of life that relate to psychological well-being. Understanding the reality of life is beneficial for individuals who lose the meaning of life because of their painful experiences. The loneliness epidemic that happened in many developed countries has resulted in a psychological problem of emptiness, and a lack of meaning and purpose of life. These people are losing their hope for the future because they do not have a comprehensive understanding of the dynamics of life and because their experiences are not in accordance with their expectations. When we comprehend the reality of human life in a wider perspective, this kind of feeling can be prevented. Understanding the wider perspective of life can be also used as an approach in tazkiya therapy. The seven realities of life will be explained in the following sections.

Life is a journey from Alláh to Alláh

As already mentioned in the introduction, life in this world is actually a journey from Alláh to Alláh. As always, one of the characteristics of a journey is that there will be challenges. Life is full of challenges, and that is undeniable. The failure to comprehend these facts will result in disappointment, frustration and depression. According to Moneim (2018), there are two categories of challenges: external challenges and internal challenges. The ability to comprehend these challenges and accept them as a reality will provide the foundation for psychological health and a form of peaceful heart.

According to the Qur'ân, there are two fundamental roles that human beings play while they are on this journey in the world. The first role is as *Khalifa*, which means that human beings have a mission to perform in this world. In general, there are five missions of human beings in this world that relate to five relations. The first relation is with Alláh, and human beings are supposed to worship Alláh in their heart, all the time. The second mission concerns the relationship with nature. Human beings have the mission to take care of nature and the environment as their place to live in this world. Nature is very important for the well-being of human beings, and it also acts as the

DOI: 10.4324/9781032717340-2

source of wisdom and human knowledge. In the Qur'ânic term, the universe or nature has the same root word as knowledge. That is why the universe is actually the source of knowledge. The third relation is with other human beings. The mission be performed in this context is to learn from each other and to collaborate in order to build a better society that will provide protection for the well-being of everyone. The fourth relation concerns man-made things, including wealth, technology and other equipment that make life easier to live. The mission concerning this relation is that human beings should be the master, and this thing should serve human needs. This would be encouraged when human beings treat these things as if they are the purpose of life. The fifth relation, which is the most fundamental in this context, is the relationship to the human self. The mission that has to be performed is tazkiya; this means that all human beings have the mission to always purify, nourish and grow themselves to become better people throughout their lives.

In order to perform these missions, human beings should never forget that all of these missions should be done for the sake of complying with Alláh's guidance. These reflect the second role of human beings when they live in this world. The second role is as *Abdullah*, which means the servant of Alláh who has to always comply with the guidance from Alláh. These two roles have to be performed simultaneously so that human beings can be effective and also safe from psychological problems. In chapter 2, verse 38, of the Qur'ân, it is

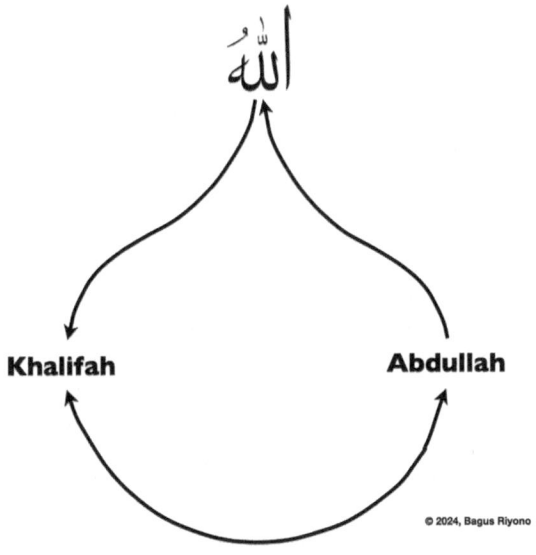

3

Figure 2.1 Life as a journey from Alláh to Alláh (Theory 1)

mentioned that those who follow and comply with a loss guidance will not experience fear or sadness.

- *We said, "Descend all of you! Then when guidance comes to you from Me, whoever follows it, there will be no fear for them, nor will they grieve."*

[Al Baqarah (2):38]

Heart is the core of human self

Based on the Qur'ânic messages and Hadith of Rasulullah (☻), the heart is the core of human self. This understanding also inspired the basic framework of Al-Ghazali's work, the *Ihya Ulumuddin*. Actually, this understanding about the heart is also part of the European and Asian civilisations and culture that can be found in the classic literature. For example when someone memorises something, the English expression is to know by heart. The Greek word for heart is "cardia," which means the core of human beings. In Eastern culture, for example Japanese, the word for heart is "kokoro," and "kokoro" is always in the heart of Japanese culture. We can find this phenomenon in every culture if we explore further.

Conventional psychology unfortunately has not reached this understanding of the heart. The state-of-the-art psychological research is still focused on the brain. This means that conventional psychology has not reached the reality of human life concerning the heart. On the other hand, psychology that was developed from an Islāmic perspective, for example that developed by Al-Ghazali in the eleventh century, has understood these realities since the beginning.

Tazkiya therapy is a psychological approach based on the Islāmic perspective, so it continues the worldview of Imam Al-Ghazali and his contemporaries. If we study brain science carefully from a brain expert, we will find evidence that the brain actually is not the place of the human mind. Some evidence revealed by neurosurgeons showed that whatever they did to the brain does not significantly influence individual personality and their minds (Sperry, 1968; Eccles, 1994). Neuroscientists also argue that something at the quantum level controls the brain. Eccles (1994) called it the self or the soul. In the Qur'ânic term, the soul is the *nafs*, and the heart is the core of the soul. So, from the Islāmic perspective, the soul and the heart cannot be separated.

As already mentioned in the Introduction, dealing with the heart is not the same as dealing with the brain. The brain is a part of the human organ that is material in nature, and it can be divided, for example, between the left hemisphere and the right hemisphere. When we deal with the heart, we cannot divide it into parts. The heart is immaterial and is a part of the unseen reality that has different characteristics from the brain. The heart is the one that understands, the one that makes decisions and the one that can bring the self

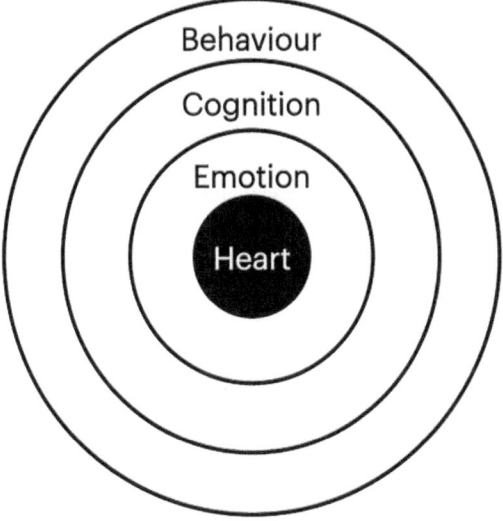

Figure 2.2 Heart as the core of human beings (Theory 2)

towards a better or worse condition. The heart is the one that will determine the individual who has psychological health or psychological problems.

Understanding the reality that the core of human beings is the heart will help the client and the therapist to focus on the cause of any psychological problem. The faculties of the human heart include the ability to reason, the capacity to empathise and the sensitivity of the conscience. These three faculties are the ones that can cause psychological problems and the key to regain psychological health.

This understanding of the reality of the human heart is very important for tazkiya therapy because this is one of the fundamentals that differentiate tazkiya therapy from other psychotherapies. By focusing on the heart, the process of tazkiya therapy will explore the cause of any psychological problems. If the approach of the cognitive behaviour therapy (CBT) focuses on thinking about the consequences and the benefit of behaviour, tazkiya therapy also explores the reason why the client chooses to behave in a particular way. In other words, since the heart is an unseen reality, it is not contained or limited in time and space so that what has been happening in the past is actually also present and influences the current condition of the heart. Other than that, the depth of the person's consciousness, how they understand the reality, is also another dimension of the heart that is also responsible for the current condition of the heart.

Here is one example of these multidimensional dynamics of the heart. An individual currently has a problem of anxiety. He/she is anxious about the future of his/her career. This anxiety grows after the individual observes the changes that happen so fast in the workforce that make him/her unsure whether he/she can compete in an always changing environment. He/she defines success in career as a prerequisite of happiness. This example shows that there are at least two dimensions that are happening simultaneously in the heart that cause this anxiety. If he/she can switch the belief about happiness, the anxiety can also disappear. For example, if happiness is defined as the result of caring for or helping others, and it does not have anything to do with career success, there is no need to be anxious about the ever-changing environment and the unclear career future.

A metaphor of one individual who has a psychological problem is a house on fire. When a house is on fire, what people see from a distance is that there is a lot of smoke coming from that house. This smoke is the metaphor of the behaviour, something that is observable from a distance. To solve this problem of house on fire is not just to get rid of the smoke. Even though you can use a very big fan to blow the smoke away, the problem will still persist. This smoke is just the consequence of the fire in the house that is not observable from outside. This fire is a metaphor of the heart. If you want to solve the problem, what you have to do is extinguish the fire inside the house, meaning you have to enter the house and find where the fire is. When you are approaching the fire, you can feel the heat first before you finally find the fire itself. This heat is the metaphor of emotion and cognition. This means that to understand what is going on with the heart, sometimes we have to go through emotional turmoil or rationalisation from the client. Rationalisation is a form of defence mechanism, so they have excuses not to reveal the actual problem. A tazkiya therapist should be aware of emotional turmoil and rationalisation so that they can comprehend the core problem that is in the heart of the client. In order to do so, first of all, the therapist should gain trust, so the client can feel comfortable to say the truth.

There are four basic potentials of the human heart

All human beings have four basic potentials that relate to the capacity of the heart. These potentials are endowed by Alláh for every individual to develop them. Potential is a modality that can be developed but also will be idle if the individual does not intentionally develop them. These potentials are sensing, reasoning, empathy and conscience (Riyono, 2023).

These potentials can also be called as the faculties of the heart. There are four faculties of the human heart. The first faculty, which is the most superficial, is sensory in nature. This faculty is illustrated as the outermost layer of the soul, and it is called sensing potential. There are five senses that humans have, which are hearing, sight, smell, touch and taste. There are two sensing potentials that have a significant role in psychological health: hearing and sight. Hearing is the capability to process knowledge from narrative resources. Sight is the capability to acquire knowledge from witnessing events or incidents in life. Both hearing and sight are faculties of the heart to gain understanding of the environment or oneself through knowledge. In this case, when we talk about hearing and sight, we are not talking about ears and eyes, but the whole system of hearing and sight that involves the ears, the eyes and the nervous system; the chemical and the electrical parts of the nervous system and the process of understanding, which happens in the heart. There is a verse in the Qur'ân that criticises those who have ears but do not listen and have eyes but can't see (Al-A'râf (7):179). Therefore, the faculty of sensing is actually one of the human potentials that can be developed to become more effective in developing knowledge and wisdom.

- *And We have certainly created for Hell many of the jinn and mankind. They have hearts with which they do not understand, they have eyes with which they do not see, and they have ears with which they do not hear. Those are like livestock; rather, they are more astray. It is they who are the heedless.*

[Al-A'râf (7):179]

The second faculty of the heart is called reasoning. Reasoning is the capability to process an information that is obtained from the sensing process to become reasonable knowledge that complies with logic, connects to the purpose and develops a meaning. Reasoning deals with ideas, concepts and other abstract information. In other words, reasoning represents the human capability of abstraction. Reasoning deals with abstract concepts from the environment and from within the self. Reasoning will answer the questions "why," "what," "how" and "what for." In the classic work of Muslim scholars, the term used for reasoning is *'aql*. However, some contemporary scholars separate *'aql* from *nafs* and *qalb*. This separation sometimes causes confusion and is not quite accurate if we revert to the Qur'ânic messages. In the study of the Qur'ânic narration, actually *'aql* or reasoning is not a separate entity from the heart and the soul, but rather it is the faculty of the heart, or it can be said that *'aql* is the function of the heart.

The question about "who" or "others" in terms of relationship will be explained by the third faculty of the heart, which is empathy. Empathy is the human faculty that involves emotion and the meaning of interpersonal relationships. Empathy also connects with the sensing faculty in a way that the process of obtaining information about "who" is done by sensing as well. Empathy is not the same as reasoning because the core characteristic of empathy involves emotion, while reasoning is more involved with cognition. However, reasoning and empathy don't work separately, so there are also interactions between the two; for example, when the emotion becomes excessive, the reasoning can be neutralised by contemplating the purpose and the reason having the excessive emotion. It also helps the emotion to become less excessive after some deliberate contemplation.

The fourth faculty, which is the deepest in the heart, is called conscience. Conscience is the faculty of the heart that connects to Alláh and all the reality beyond the physical worlds. Conscience is the capability of the human soul to see and understand the bigger picture of human life beyond the life in this world, which involves the Hereafter, the heaven and the hell, and also about the angels and the devils. The understanding of the existence of the angels and the devils in our day-to-day lives will provide an individual with the attitude of heedfulness. The existence of angels and devils can be felt by every individual, whether they believe it or not. Those who don't believe in angels and devils use terms such as inner voice, whispers in the heart, automatic thinking, unconscious desire and altered state of consciousness. The theories of psychology actually have noticed these phenomena, but they attribute these to something that is unclear, such as in the transpersonal approach about altered state of consciousness (Valverde, 2015).

A more detailed explanation of each basic human potential is as follows.

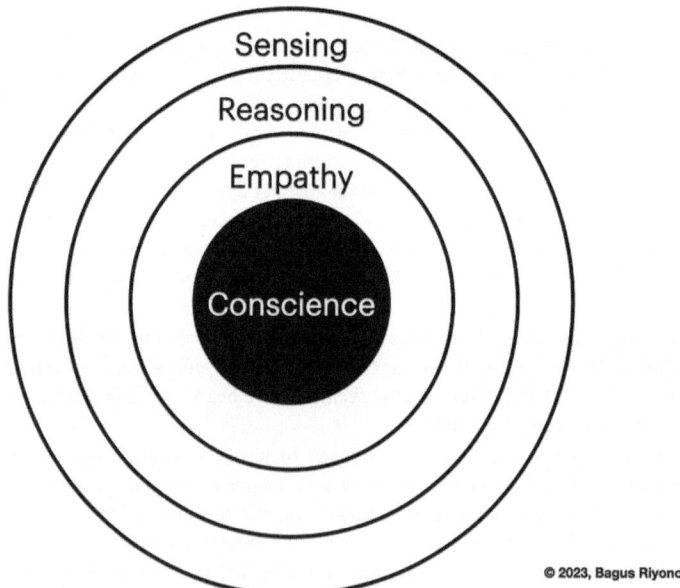

© 2023, Bagus Riyono

Figure 2.3 Theory of the layers of the human soul (Theory 3)

Sensing

Sensing is the outermost potential of the soul that is directly connected to the body. In other words, sensing is in the form of the five senses. It is like the soul as an entity that is attached to the body, with its outer shell directly attached to the body. Sensing is really feeling something concrete, that is here and now, that can be seen, heard, touched, smelled and even tasted if necessary.

Reasoning

The deeper potential of the soul is reasoning. Reasoning potential includes something more than concrete objects. This potential has entered an abstract space. When someone uses reasoning, they can see something deeper than what is detected by the senses. He can describe an abstract concept. When the reasoning is active, an individual can understand the reason of what is happening and also the consequences that are not yet detected by the sensing. Reasoning can also construct meaning of the issue that is experienced by the individual.

Reasoning is able to process something that is observed and felt, more than just describing. In this dimension, there is a causal relationship, there is a reason, there is a purpose and there is meaning. If sensing is a connection between the soul and the body, reasoning is a connection between the soul and the signs that make humans understand more about the meaning of human life. People who have trouble with reasoning will not understand any explanations. In other words, for people who live but are unable to explain, who do not have reasons for the actions they have committed, it could be that the reasoning potential in their souls has not been well developed.

Reasoning will stimulate the formation of meaning in a person in interpreting what that person is experiencing. However, it should be understood that the meaning generated by individuals is not always correct because the rumination process can produce false meanings. According to Riyono (2020), false meaning is something that seems as if it is a meaning, but it is not the real meaning and tends to deceive and cause disappointment. False meaning is short-term, self-centred, illusory and driven by revenge or superficial understanding. On the other hand, true meaning includes a sense of contribution, a sense of competence, a sense of enjoyment and a sense of values (Riyono, 2020).

Empathy

The potential of the soul that is deeper than reasoning is known as empathy. Empathy is not just a feeling. Empathy is the connection between one's soul and another's soul. In general, empathy for individuals encourages behaviour that supports social relations. Thus, it is true that empathy is deeper than reasoning. True love is love that activates the level of empathy from one's soul with another. A certain group of people only talk about love at the level of sensing, so they don't differentiate between love and sexual relations. In the discourse of conventional psychology, this view is supported by the theory of Freud who put forward the concept of the "Id", which is referred to as the source of sexual libido. Meanwhile, Maslow (1970a) included love in the category of social needs. Maslow differentiated between love and sex; that is, he put sexual need as part of the physiological needs. Besides love, empathy also represents the capacity for compassion for the suffering of others.

Conscience

The deepest potential of the soul is conscience, which is spiritual in nature. Conscience is the potential that is closest to the existence of the spirit, namely the connection between the soul and God which shows the human longing for God. An indicator of a strongly developed conscience is the consciousness about the relationship with Alláh and the belief of Hereafter. This level of consciousness is the source of endless hope, which is the most important element in human motivation.

These potentials will become human consciousness that varies among individuals. The deeper the consciousness, the stronger the personality will be. The most superficial level of consciousness is the sensing mentality. This happens when the individual has not put enough effort to develop reasoning, empathy and conscience. When the level of consciousness is only the sensing layer, the individual will have not enough reasons and will behave only based on sensation or impulse. Sensing mentality is the most severe condition of consciousness. The individual who has a sensing mentality also lacks empathy and usually feels emptiness in the heart because they do not have a strong enough awareness of meaning. It does not mean they do not have reasoning, empathy and conscience but that they have not developed them properly. Some other individuals might already develop reasoning potential and can behave reasonably. However, this is not enough because when they do not develop empathy, they will face problems when interacting with other people. An individual whose consciousness is limited at the level of reasoning will only care about their ideas and their arguments that sometimes do not benefit other people around them. Empathy is very important to prevent antisocial behaviour. The most severe psychological disorder when the empathy potential does not develop is sociopathy.

When an individual already develops sensing, reasoning and empathy, they will become humanist. They will be able to adjust and have healthy interactions with other people. In the perspective of conventional psychology, this individual will be considered to have mental health. The term used to illustrate this individual is a "fully functioning person."

From the perspective of humanistic psychology, a fully functioning person is an individual who has already attained effectiveness in social life. This effectiveness in a social relation also covers the issues of morality and tolerance. However, morality from the humanistic perspective does not relate to God. That's why according to Maslow (1970b), morality is relative to the culture. Different cultures will have different moral standards. At this point, the Islāmic perspective does not totally agree with the moral relativity, even though the Qur'ân recognises the cultural differences. The Qur'ân respects differences of the culture, but more than that there is a universal morality in the Islāmic teaching that relates to Alláh. This is mentioned in Surah Al-Hujurat (49):13.

- *humanity! Indeed, We created you from a male and a female, and made you into peoples and tribes so that you may "get to" know one another. Surely the most noble of you in the sight of Allah is the most righteous among you. Allah is truly All-Knowing, All-Aware.*

[Al-Hujurat (49):13]

According to Riyono (2023), cultural morality is represented by empathy, while universal morality is represented by the conscience. From the perspective of tazkiya therapy, empathy alone is not sufficient. The one who has optimum psychological health is the one who also develops the conscience, so that the level of consciousness is deep enough to realise the unseen reality of human life. This is important because no human beings can escape death. Only those who have already developed the conscience are the ones who are ready to face death. If the conscience is not well developed, death will become a terror in their heart. In the literature of conventional psychology, there is a term called terror management (Greenberg & Arndt, 2012).

Unfortunately, this terror management issue is not aimed to awaken or develop the conscience potential of individuals but rather to help them forget about death so that they will not be terrorised by it. Therefore, the concept of terror management does not align with the reality of human life. An individual cannot develop the conscience by themselves. This is the part where Alláh's role is needed because only Alláh can switch the heart from unbelieving to believing. The effort that can be made to achieve this is limited to suggest the client to open their heart for Alláh's guidance.

In tazkiya therapy, these phenomena can be explained in multidimensional ways. The influence of angels and devils is one dimension of these phenomena, but there is also the energy of the self that can invoke these phenomena. The four layers of the soul (sensing, reasoning, empathy and conscience) are the source of energy that will ignite human freedom. For example, when someone sees that a woman is beaten by a man in a park, the human freedom is ignited so that the individual can choose what action he/she will conduct, whether it is to help the woman or act as if he/she didn't see it. In this example, the sensing layer is active in terms of seeing someone beaten, the reasoning layer is active in terms of knowing that someone is in danger and the empathy layer is active in terms of feeling that someone needs help. However, the quality of the conscience layer can influence him/her through his/her motive to help or not. In other words, human freedom is actually a product that is the internal energy of the human soul, which is quite complex. This freedom will manifest in human behaviour. When the individual has behavioural and/ or emotional problems, there are three forces that cause these to happen. The first cause is the human potential in the form of sensing, reasoning, empathy and conscience. The second force is the influence of angels and devils that imposes good or bad ideas for the self that is mediated by four basic human potentials. The third force is the environmental influence that is internalised by the individual through the four faculties of the heart.

Adding to those forces that influence human behaviour, there is also one negative force within the human part, which in Arabic terms is called *hawwa*. *Hawwa* is a negative energy of the self that can corrupt the human potential so that it will cause problematic behaviour. For example, this negative energy of the self can be in the form of laziness, ignorance, excessive desires, anger, and so forth. Satanic influence will provoke this negative energy so that it becomes excessive and can be manifested in a behaviour. This satanic temptation can be in the form of rationalisation, excuses, illusion and deception so that the self will feel good to follow this negative energy. On the other hand, the angels will counter this negative energy with reasonable thought, reminding the individual of the purpose and the meaning that they should achieve in their lives. If the conscience is strong, then the individual will follow the influence of the angels, but if the conscience is weak, the individual will follow the satanic temptation. This is what freedom is all about, which can bring goodness and also have the risk to bring wickedness.

The most important function to strengthen the conscience is to connect with Alláh the Almighty because we cannot escape from satanic temptation without help from Alláh. The satanic temptation can become the source of psychological problems. The psychological problem that is caused by satanic temptation will be more severe than the problem of cognition, emotion and behaviour. This means that if the psychological problems are caused by the individual's inability to get away from the satanic temptation, the emotion, cognition and behaviour will be also influenced and will be disturbed. On the other hand, once the conscience is well-developed, and the connection with Alláh becomes stronger, the individual will be protected from any psychological problem.

Human beings are motivated by meaning

There is something that cannot be denied about human beings. All or every individual has the capacity to choose and decide how they will think, feel and behave. This reality explains why there are individual differences in human beings. The other side of the reality about human beings is that every individual has something that they claim to be meaningful for themselves. The diversity of meaning among individuals is driven by their freedom to choose and inspired by the level of consciousness. This reality relates closely to the third reality explained above. To find meaning for something that is meaningful is very logical and natural for all human beings. However, beyond this diverse meaning that each individual can choose, there is a true meaning that is guided by the optimum level of consciousness.

A true meaning is something that is universal and eternal and undeniable. However, because of the different levels of consciousness that each individual has, not everybody can instantly understand what these true meanings are. For example, those who focus on gaining and collecting material possession in their life might perceive that the highest meaning of life is material possession. A lot of people have these perceptions of meaning. They always measure success by material benefit.

Another group of people might perceive power as the highest meaning of life. If an individual thinks this way, they will exert extra effort to gain power or to be a powerful person, whether in the family community or nationwide or maybe the entire world. It is not so difficult to understand

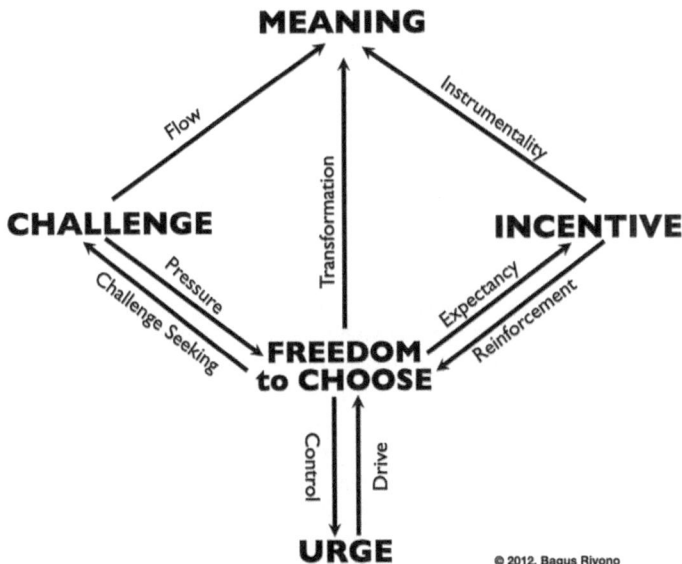

© 2012, Bagus Riyono

Figure 2.4 Theory of meaning (Theory 4)

that the urge to gain power and the urge to increase material possession are sometimes intertwined. Some people might be driven by ambition to gain power so that they can have a lot of material possession. On the other hand, some other people might ambitiously pursue wealth so that they can have power based on the abundance of their material possessions. Both cases have a false meaning.

The true meaning relates to the first reality that eventually everybody will die and leave this world to meet Alláh in the Hereafter. So true meaning is anything that is derived from the understanding of the first reality. It could be in the form of acquiring knowledge for the betterment of humanity or participating in social works to help people in need and anything that is coherent in this path.

Besides freedom to choose, individuals also have another psychological force in the form of urge. Urge consists of four dynamics: revenge, wants, needs and instinct. Instinct is the behaviour that will automatically happen when an individual needs to survive from a critical event. The critical situation might happen when there is a fire, a natural disaster or a life-threatening incident. Needs is the basic requirement for individuals to be able to survive, for example food, water and settlement. Wants is something that an individual thinks they should have but actually is not always necessary. As long as it is reasonable, wants can benefit individuals to progress in their life. However, when what they want is something that is unreasonable, it will cause psychological problems. Revenge is the energy that responds to bad experiences in the past. This bad experience can be disappointment, broken heart, traumatic events, feeling hurt because someone has done bad things to an individual, guilt or shame. When an individual has revenge in their heart, they will not have inner peace. What is represented by revenge is part of the disease in the heart that has to be purified.

Life is a test in the form of uncertainties

The keyword of these life challenges is uncertainty. Every individual from any cultural background or any country in the world is always facing uncertainties in their life. Any effort and any activities that any individuals do are trying to close the gap of uncertainty. When we make a plan, what we really do is avoid uncertainty as much as possible. But nobody can avoid uncertainty totally because this is the reality of human life in this world. There is a literature in psychology that studies uncertainty and mental health. The final conclusion is that the root of any psychological problem is intolerance of uncertainty (Yuaniardi et al., 2017). Uncertainty is not something to be avoided, but it is something to tolerate. Meaning that what we have to do is to accept that the reality of life is uncertain, but we need to do something to keep it at the level that we can tolerate.

Some concepts that relate to uncertainty are risk and hope, challenge and opportunity, and also possibilities. Risk is the probability of bad things that could happen out of uncertainty. That is why anything we do in our life is to minimise risk. Hope is the possibility of good things that could happen out of uncertainty. Hope can become a psychological power that plays as the protective factor for psychological health. Hope is defined as belief that beyond uncertainty there will be something good (Riyono, 2012). Challenge is the other side of uncertainty that we have to go through in order to fulfil our needs. On the other hand, opportunity is something good that we can pursue in the universe of uncertainty. Possibilities are the variety of conditions that we should be prepared to accept as the result of our effort. The ability to accept possibilities and move on to other possibilities is one of the characteristics of psychologically healthy individuals.

The interplay among risk, uncertainty and hope will result in five psychological states: (1) the psychological state of learned helplessness, (2) psychological state of optimum challenge, (3) the psychological state of fatalism, (4) optimum opportunity and (5) comfort zone.

Psychological states of learned helplessness (Seligman, 1972) happen when the risk reaches the maximum and hope is minimum. This psychological state is experienced by individuals who have been experiencing multiple failures in their life and have a negative mindset about themselves and about the future. This psychological state is happening in individuals who suffer from frustration or depression. When this happens, the approach to heal is to instil hope in their heart.

The second psychological state is called optimum challenge. The psychological state of optimum challenge happens when individuals see a little hope above uncertainty, but the pressure is quite strong. At this state, the individual will feel a strong challenge to cope with. Usually, in this condition, an individual will have extra energy to jump out of the problem, but the energy is not

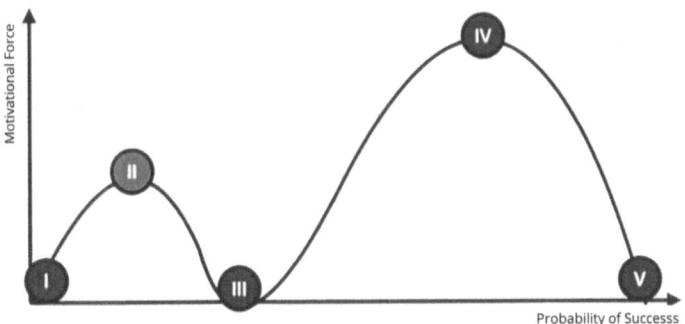

Figure 2.5 Five psychological states (Theory 5)

sustainable. The example of this state is when an individual faces a critical situation and has to act quickly to avoid the risk of the situation, for example when an individual is trapped in a fire. Another example is when an individual has to finish a test at the last minute. For some instances, the psychological state might bring up some extraordinary results that are surprising. However, this condition is not reliable because there is too much risk. If an individual has a custom with a psychological state of optimum challenge, they will always live in a crisis situation. This will drain the psychological resources of the individual. They feel tired psychologically, and at the end, they might experience burn out. There is why, even though some surprising result will happen, the psychological state of optimum challenge is not an ideal condition. This condition is also prone to anxiety disorder.

The third psychological state is the psychological state of fatalism. This happens when an individual has a mindset that everything happened by chance. When this psychological state is experienced by an individual, they will become ignorant, lazy and not motivated to do anything, but they will tend to blame others if bad things happen to them. If this psychological state stays, then an individual will always complain about life, and they will eventually have a negative attitude towards anything. This attitude will create problems in individuals' relationships with other people, such as with spouse, family and co-workers.

The fourth psychological state is optimum opportunity, which is the ideal state that tazkiya therapy tries to achieve. The psychological state of optimum opportunity is the most realistic attitude towards the dynamics about life that will make an individual calm but yet have the energy to live an active and meaningful life. The characteristics of this psychological state are as follows. Firstly, they have a strong hope for the future, meaning that they always believe that there will be opportunities in every situation. This hope becomes the source of energy for the individual to move on with their life happily and strongly motivated. Secondly, the individual in this psychological state of optimum opportunity tolerates uncertainty, in a way that they are aware of the possibilities that could happen, but these possibilities do not make them anxious. The third characteristic of the individual is they are always aware of the risk of any action, so they are always prepared for the worst and are cautious in their step forwards.

The fifth psychological state, the psychological state of a comfort zone, happens when an individual has very high confidence in their abilities and their future. This mindset is deceiving because the reality of life is full of uncertainty that anything could happen to anyone beyond their imagination. Individuals who have the psychological state of comfort zone expect that they will always be successful and that the situation will always be in control. Expectation is very strong in these individuals. They do not tolerate mistakes, and they do not accept uncertainty. When everything is normal, it seems that this individual does not have problems. However, when the situation changes in a bad way, those who have a psychological state of comfort zone will be surprised and cannot accept the reality. When this happens, they will become frustrated, and it is going to be difficult for them to stand up again. They will see this unexpected condition as the end of the world. Some cases of this phenomenon ended with suicide. For example, some students experience high achievement like becoming top students of the class from kindergarten until high school; when these students enter the university, they become surprised by the challenges that they never imagined before. Some instances of such cases ended up in suicide.

Learning from the phenomenon of the psychological state of comfort zone, we have to understand the big difference between hope and expectation. Hope is a protective factor for psychological health, while expectation is a risk factor for psychological health. Hope makes an individual able to tolerate uncertainties, but expectation does the contrary. When what we have is expectation, we demand that everything should happen in accordance with our expectations. When things go wrong, individuals with expectations will be very disappointed. On the other hand, individuals with hope realise and accept that life is full of uncertainty; whatever happens, whether it is good or bad, will not break their heart. Hope is always alive in any situation or condition because hope is a belief that is intrinsic in nature, so it is not affected by the environmental conditions. Expectation, on the other hand, is extrinsic in nature because it demands the environment to satisfy the individual. These differences are very fundamental, and tazkiya therapists have to be sensitive to opposite psychological forces that seem to be similar.

Human beings are vulnerable

The sixth reality of life is that human beings are actually vulnerable. Compared to wild beasts, human beings are weak. Human beings also easily get sick. Sometimes human beings become helpless because of a very tiny virus that infects the body. Another reality of vulnerability is that human beings are forgetful and cannot beat the computer in retrieving memories or information. Human beings are also very vulnerable when facing natural disasters. Human life can easily be taken away because of floods, earthquakes and volcanic eruptions. These facts defy that human beings actually are vulnerable. Human beings also need each other to have psychological and social support in their life.

Naturally to compensate for these vulnerabilities, human beings usually have anchors to rely on. There are four categories of anchors that an individual can rely on to compensate for their vulnerabilities.

The first anchor is others. Since a baby, actually all individuals need other people to take care of them and to help them survive. When they become independent, they will add another anchor, which is self. This is called self-reliance. From the perspective of human development, the third anchor that

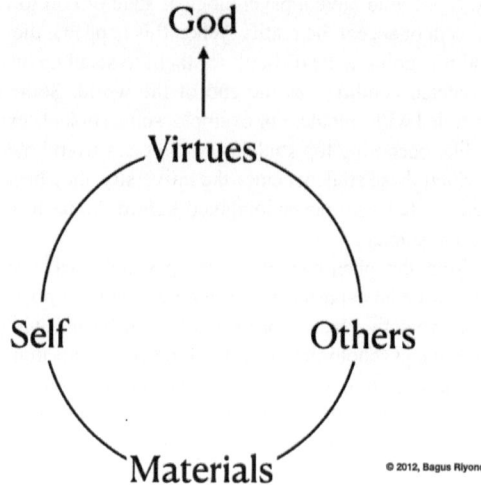

Figure 2.6 Theory of anchor (Theory 6)

developed when a person is already settled in his life is material possession. This means that besides depending on others and themselves, they start to utilise their wealth as the source for satisfaction and happiness.

The ideal characteristic of an anchor is reliability. Since an anchor is something that is needed to compensate for human vulnerability, when it becomes unreliable, it will create psychological problems. These three anchors, materials, self and others, are not always reliable. Others can betray you, and you can become sick and weak. And materials are very easy to disappear. That is why these three anchors are not enough to guarantee stability. The fourth anchor is called virtues. Virtue is something that is material and conceptual in nature, but since it has the characteristic of universality and eternity, it is more reliable than the other three anchors. According to Aristòteles (2001), "A virtue is a trait of excellence, including traits that may be moral, social, or intellectual." In Qur'ânic terms, virtues represent *hikmah* or wisdom. When an individual anchor is virtues, they will always be able to rely on that because virtues are universal and eternal. This means that anchoring to virtues is the prescription for psychological health.

Freedom, uncertainty and vulnerability always coexist in every moment of human life

There are three laws of human life that will be explained in this section based on the synthesis of the previous theoretical frameworks. These three laws

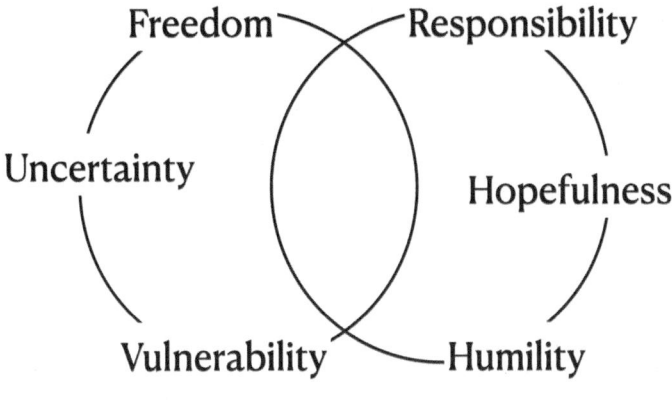

Figure 2.7 Law of human life (Theory 7)

involve three pairs of stimulus–response-like relationships. These laws are not three independent laws, but they are three dimensions of human life that are simultaneously experienced by every individual. By understanding these laws of human life, an individual will be able to manage life effectively.

The tazkiya therapy approach to instil hope can be done by stimulating the reasoning that will give the client a broader perspective of the future with possibilities. The second approach can be done by providing psychological support to the client as a way to strengthen their empathy and compassion and to remind the client about their loved ones that they always need their presence to support them. The third approach in tazkiya therapy to heal this psychological condition is to remind them about the reality of life as a journey that needs to be finished so that they can enter the next life with a happy and released feeling (Figures 2.1–2.7).

References

Aristòteles. (2001). *Ètica a nicòmaco*. Alianza Editorial.

Eccles, J. C. (1994). *How the self controls its brain*. Springer.

Greenberg, J., & Arndt, J. (2012). Terror management theory. *Handbook of Theories of Social Psychology*, *1*, 398–415.

Maslow, A. H. (1970a). *Motivation and personality* (2nd ed.). Harper and Row.

Maslow, A. H. (1970b). New introduction: Religions, values, and peak-experiences. *Journal of Transpersonal Psychology*, *2*(2), 83–90.

Moneim, A. A. (2018). Towards Islāmic Maqasidi education philosophy for sustainable development: Qur'ânic perspective with special attention to Indonesia, *17*(2), 221–266. https//doi/:10.20885/millah.vol17.iss2.art4

Riyono, B. (2020). *Motivasi dan kepribadian: perspektif islam tentang dinamika jiwa dan perilaku manusia.* Al-Mawardi Prima.

Riyono, B. (2023). Constructing the theory of human basic potential based on Qur'ânic Messages: Study with Maqasid methodology. *Minbar Islāmic Studies, 16*(2), 449–475. https://doi.org/10.31162/2618-9569-2023-16-2-449-475

Riyono, B., & Himam, F. (2012). In search for anchors the fundamental motivational force in compensating for human vulnerability. *Gadjah Mada International Journal of Business, 14*(3), 229–252. https://doi.org/10.22146/gamaijib.5475

Seligman, M. E. (1972). Learned helplessness. *Annual Review of Medicine, 23*(1), 407–412. https://doi.org/10.1146/annurev.me.23.020172.002203

Sperry, R. W. (1968). Hemisphere deconnection and unity in conscious awareness. *American Psychologist, 23*(10), 723.

The Noble Qur'ân Encyclopedia. (n.d.). *English translation – Saheeh International.* https://quranenc.com/en/browse/english_saheeh

Valverde, R. (2015). Neurotechnology as a tool for inducing and measuring altered states of consciousness in transpersonal psychotherapy. *NeuroQuantology, 13*(4), 1–16. https://doi.org/10.14704/nq.2015.13.4.870

Yuniardi, M. S., Freeston, M. H., & Rodgers, J. (2017). *Intolerance of uncertainty, social anxiety and alcohol use among students in the United Kingdom and Indonesia.* Newcastle University.

3   Seven indicators of psychological health

The concept of psychological health based on Qur'ânic teaching is not limited to comfort, adjustment, joyfulness, acceptance and so on. The concept of psychological health will include struggle, sacrifice, restrain and other conditions that an individual has to go through as part of a test in life.

A healthy soul is a soul that is peaceful, solid, full, balanced, coherent, resilient and ever-growing. These indicators are the condition of the heart. As mentioned earlier, the concept of psychological health is more comprehensive than mental health. The following seven indicators reflect the condition of the heart that eventually influences the mind, the emotion and the spirituality of the individual.

A peaceful heart

The ultimate indicator of psychological health is a peaceful heart. In the Al-Qur'ân, there are several verses that mention a peaceful heart in various expressions. The first one is *nafs al-muthmainnah*, which means a peaceful soul. Again, in the Al-Qur'ân, the heart (*qalb*) and the soul (*nafs*) are interchangeably used and refer to the individual self. Sometimes, the term chest (*shudur*) is also used to refer to the heart. We have to understand that the Al-Qur'ân referring to this issue is something that is immaterial. Something that is unseen and unobservable but can be detected through contemplation or feeling. In this case, the term heart will be used for the purposes of practicality and ease of understanding.

Another term on the Al-Qur'ân concerning a peaceful heart is *qalbun salim*. *Salim* also means peaceful. Another expression about a peaceful heart is *tathmainnu al-qulub*, which combined *muthmainnah* and *qalb* in an active way.

- *those who believe and whose hearts find comfort in the remembrance of Allah. Surely in the remembrance of Allah do hearts find comfort.* [Ar-Ra'd (13):28]

DOI: 10.4324/9781032717340-3

- *Allah will say to the righteous, "O tranquil soul! Return to your Lord, well pleased with Him and well pleasing to Him. So join My servants, and enter My Paradise.*

[Al-Fajr (89):27–30]

Three of these conditions of the heart are related to Alláh and Heaven (*jannah*). Therefore, the ultimate indicator of psychological health is anchored to Alláh and the Hereafter. We can explore more about this peaceful heart with at least two keywords, that is belief in Alláh and the Hereafter, and this is mentioned in Surah Al-Baqarah (2):62.

- *whoever truly believes in Allah and the Last Day and does good will have their reward with their Lord. And there will be no fear for them, nor will they grieve.*

[Al-Baqarah (2):62]

This teaches us that the key to psychological health is remembering Alláh and the orientation to the Hereafter. This indicator is related to the first reality that life is a journey from Alláh to Alláh.

From the messages in Surah Al-Baqarah (2):62 above, we found the notion that a peaceful heart is the heart that "has no fear for them, nor will they grieve." Fear in the psychological term relates to anxiety, and grief relates to depression. It means that anxiety and depression are diseases of the heart that make it unpeaceful.

Besides believing in Alláh and the Hereafter, an individual also needs to do good deeds because a human being is social in nature. In the Qur'ânic term, there are at least two dimensions of human relation: the first is the relation to Alláh (*hablun mina-Alláh*), and the second is the relation to other human beings (*hablun mina an-nas*). Since human relation has two dimensions, to achieve a peaceful heart, an individual should work in these two dimensions simultaneously. Believing in Alláh and the Hereafter is what an individual should do from the first dimension, and doing good deeds is another thing that all individuals should do in the social dimension. This guidance is also strongly mentioned in the Qur'ân Surah Al-'Asr (103):1–3.

- *By the passage of time! Surely humanity is in grave loss, except those who have faith, do good, and urge each other to the truth, and urge each other to perseverance.*

[Al-'Asr (103):1–3]

At the end of Surah Al-Asr, it is mentioned there are two principles of good deeds, which is to be truthful (*haq*) and to be patient (*shabr*). These two principles will be elaborated further in six additional indicators to achieve a peaceful heart.

A peaceful heart is the ultimate indicator of psychological health that can be achieved through certain discipline. In this book, there are six additional indicators that reflect six disciplines for achieving a peaceful heart. These six indicators are derived from the principles of truthfulness (*al-haq*) and patience (*as-shabr*). The six indicators are a (1) solid heart, (2) full heart, (3) coherent heart, (4) balanced heart, (5) resilient heart and (6) ever-growing heart.

A solid heart

Solid means not "cracked" or broken, which means free from resentment and heartache, as well as long-lasting trauma. A solid heart can also mean a strong heart that can cope with difficulties without experiencing a broken heart. The one who has a solid heart will forgive easily and is not easily hurt. That is why one attribute of a solid heart is the heart is always willing to forgive. This is mentioned in Surah Āl-'Imrān (03):134.

- *Who spend [in the cause of Allāh] during ease and hardship and who restrain anger and who pardon the people – and Allāh loves the doers of good.*

[Āl-'Imrān (3):134]

The illustration of those who have a solid heart is also mentioned in Surah Al-Furqān (25):63:

- *And the servants of the Most Merciful are those who walk upon the earth easily, and when the ignorant address them [harshly], they say [words of] peace.*

[Al-Furqān (25):63]

This illustration of a person with a solid heart shows that this person is not easily hurt by other people's attitudes or treatment. The second part of this message shows that those who have a solid heart will also always say something nice and pray for people who tried to hurt them.

To have a solid heart, we have to exercise this behaviour and make it our habit. For example, to develop a solid heart, we should always practise forgiving others. That is why the Qur'ânic message is a command to us from Alláh, meaning that we have to follow this guidance in order to obtain a solid heart. This shows that human beings actually have a choice either to make the heart solid or to let it be fragile.

A fragile heart is a heart that is easily broken – a heart that is weak. Psychological problems could be caused by this fragile heart. Some of the issues in a psychological disorder include a broken heart, disappointment, guilt and also trauma, which can then become a post-traumatic stress disorder. The key for overcoming this psychological problem is to exercise forgiveness and to have a positive view of other human beings and also of life so that the heart will not be easily broken. The more we exercise forgiveness and hope, the stronger the heart will be.

A full heart

A full heart is the heart that is fully functioning. Full means there is no emptiness in the heart, so it avoids confusion or doubt. Feeling empty inside is another form of psychological problem that is experienced by quite a number of people. This emptiness in the heart will invoke confusion in the individual. Emptiness in the heart will also result in losing meaning in life. Individuals who have problems with the meaning of life will experience confusion and a lot of unanswered questions. This losing meaning in life can become very severe that it will invoke suicidal thoughts. When individuals lose the meaning of life, they also question the purpose of life. Suicidal thoughts come when an individual stops understanding the purpose of life. When they stop to understand the purpose of life, they will give up life. Therefore, psychological problems that concern the emptiness of the heart are very serious problems.

As we already discussed about the reality of the human soul and its four basic potentials, these serve as the faculties that connect the soul with its surroundings. These four layers of the soul are sensing, reasoning, empathy and conscience. Sensing is the connection between the soul and the surrounding, including the body and the here-and-now situation. Reasoning is the connection between a soul and ideas, concept, meaning, purpose and reason of anything that the individual is doing. Empathy is the connection between the soul and other souls. Conscience is the connection between the soul and Alláh and the Hereafter, and also other unseen realities. Emptiness of the heart happens when one or more of these layers of the soul are not functioning.

When an individual experiences loneliness, it will have an impact on the layer of empathy; in other words, loneliness is a condition when an individual is disconnected from others. This does not mean that they never meet people, but the emptiness happens because even though they meet other people every day, the heart is not connected. Therefore, loneliness is the part of the symptom concerning emptiness of the heart.

The deeper problem about this emptiness is when the conscience is not functioning properly. If this happens, the individual is disconnected from the unseen realities, which are actually the realities of the soul. When this happens, what the individual refers to themselves is only the body, and they will worry about their body because they think that their body is themselves. The effect is that this kind of emptiness can make the individual become frustrated and lose meaning as they get older and the body is not as strong as when they were younger. Individuals who suffer from this problem can also end up hurting themselves or their body. At the severe level, they can also end up committing suicide.

The cure for the issues of emptiness is to activate all the layers of the soul so that they will have a full heart. To activate reasoning, the therapist can initiate logical exercise so that the client can think more reasonably about their experiences and their problems. Reasoning can also reach out to empathy and conscience. When reasoning is activated, an individual can develop priorities that will motivate them to act accordingly. When the priority is concerning relationships with other people, it will also activate the empathy layer. However, empathy can not only be activated by reasoning but has to also be followed by experiences.

In an Islāmic tradition, a Muslim is suggested to do *silaturahim*, which means to connect to people, especially those who are closely tied to the individual. Muslims are also suggested to visit the sick ones to show care for them. These traditions are actually methods to activate empathy. Empathy can grow from understanding the importance of social interaction and experiencing interaction first hand. When reasoning and empathy are already activated, an individual can contemplate further to reach a deeper understanding of the phenomenon, and it can open the door to activate the conscience. For example, when an individual visits a friend or a family that is sick and bedridden, they will feel that actually human beings are vulnerable, and they will reason that is why human beings need Allāh the Almighty to rely on. This experience with vulnerability will also grow the attitude of humility. Usually, those who experience loneliness will feel better when they can experience these things. They will realise that their problem is actually not the worst problem that an individual could experience.

It is very important for an individual to understand and experience life in a holistic manner. As Muslims, we are commanded to always think and behave in a holistic manner because when there is an emptiness in our heart, it will be misguided by the *satan*. Al-Baqarah verse 208 states:

- *you who have believed, enter into Islām completely [and perfectly] and do not follow the footsteps of Satan. Indeed, he is to you a clear enemy.*
  [Al-Baqarah (2):208]

This Qur'ânic message implied that when there is a part of the heart that is empty, then the *satan* will infiltrate and influence the individual to the wrong direction or wrong conclusion about the situation. That is why emptiness in the heart is prone to self-harm or even suicide.

A coherent heart

The fourth indicator of psychological health is a coherent heart. Coherent means there is no conflict in the soul, and each layer supports each other and is optimally related to each other. Those who have a coherent heart are those who are protected from being hypocrites (*munafiq*). Incoherences can happen not only between the different faculties of the heart but also between the heart and the behaviour. An example of an incoherent heart is when an individual experiences emotional arousal that is not reasonable. Another example is when the faith is not coherent with the reasoning; this is also problematic, but sometimes people ignore these problems. In Islāmic teaching, reason is a very important faculty of the heart, so you have to reason about everything, including about the faith (*iman*). Islāmic faith is the most reasonable and logical faith that is always coherent in nature.

The Al-Qur'ân commands us to always use hearing, sight and intellect coherently before we do anything. In other words, what we do would be coherent with our heart based on the knowledge from our hearing and our sight. "And don't follow something you do not know. Because of hearing, sight and intellect, all of them will be held accountable." The most severe disease of the heart is the incoherence between what is in the heart and behaviour. This kind of disease is repeatedly mentioned in the Al-Qur'ân as the nature of a hypocrite. The Al-Qur'ân gives the warning that the punishment will be severe. Punishment in this case can also mean a severe psychological problem.

A balanced heart

The fifth indicator of psychological health is a balanced heart. Balanced means that each layer develops optimally, and there is no imbalance between one and the other. When the heart is imbalanced, an individual will become excessive in a certain way. For example, there are some individuals who are very rational, but they lack empathy. On the other hand, some individuals might have a strong emotion and become so emotional that sometimes they become unreasonable.

Since the human heart is very dynamic, maintaining its balance is an ongoing process. To keep the balance of the heart, an individual must have awareness about the ups and downs of their heart. This will require skills that have to be exercised continuously.

In some cases, the presence of other people is needed to remind them when they become excessive on one side of the heart. For example, when an individual becomes very emotional because something happened to someone very close to them, sometimes the emotion overrides the reason. A well-known example of this when the Prophet Muhammad (ﷺ) passed away, Umar bin Khattab became very emotional and could not accept the reality that the prophet was gone. Usually, Umar bin Khattab is known to be a rational person, but in this incident his rationality was overridden by his emotional arousal. Then, as we all know, Abu Bakar is the one who can remind Umar Bin Khattab with the following reasoning. He said, "If you worship Muhammad Rasulullah, know that Muhammad Rasulullah has passed away. But, if you worship Allāh, Allāh will live forever." This incident can happen to anyone.

That is why, when the situation is extraordinary, we need other people to remind us to keep our heart in balance.

Another case that can happen concerning this issue is that when someone is very rational and tries to explain anything with logic, sometimes they forget that there is a higher authority that might not yet be understood by his level of logic. For example, some scholars who rely too much on rational explanations cannot sometimes accept something that is beyond their ability to reason, like the existence of God. When this happens, the individual will experience severe psychological problems and will experience turbulence in their heart. This turbulence can end up in atheism. Lots of examples of atheists show that actually they previously believed in God, but when the reasoning becomes stronger and the conscience becomes weaker, they reject God. One of these people is Richard Dawkins (2016), who authored the book titled *God Delusion*. In an interview with Ben Stein, he confessed that previously he believed in God as a Christian.

In order to keep balance in our heart, first of all we have to admit that we are all vulnerable and that we do not know everything. We should also accept the reality that we are not always in control of our emotions, so sometimes we need someone to remind us. We should also always open ourselves to new knowledge and keep studying so that our perspectives will be broadened. Steve Jobs has a very valid expression about this attitude that he presented in his speech in 2005. He said that we should always "stay hungry and stay foolish," meaning we have to be hungry for new knowledge and always open our hearts because we never know everything.

A resilient heart

The sixth indicator of psychological health is a resilient heart. Resilience means being able to go through various kinds of life tests, being able to get up again when you fall, being able to return to a healthy condition when you are hurt, always being full of hope and being able to forgive yourself and others. Since life is full of dynamics, the condition of the heart is not going to be the same all the time. As implied in the term *qalb*, the heart is always changing; it will experience ups and downs along the lifespan. Nobody has a heart that is in a fixed condition all the time because everybody will always experience multilevel life tests. This certainty about life test is mentioned in Surah Al-Baqarah (2):155:

- *And We will surely test you with something of fear and hunger and a loss of wealth and lives and fruits, but give good tidings to the patient.*
  [Al-Baqarah (2):155]

At the end of this ayah, it is implied that only those who are patient can endure this test (*sabr*). Actually, the word patient cannot represent the whole meaning of *sabr* because *sabr* includes resilience and endurance besides patience. *Sabr* is a very strong psychological modality that will protect the heart from the turbulence of life tests.

As previously mentioned above, there are six indicators that will sum up a peaceful heart. A peaceful heart is not a heart that is idle or passive. A peaceful heart is a heart that is dynamic and able to always return every time it experiences some difficulties in life. Being resilient is a very important characteristic of a peaceful heart. The main attitude to ensure the resilience of the heart that will bring a peaceful condition is *sabr*. The essence of *sabr* is actually the awareness of always returning all problems experienced in life to Alláh. This characteristic of *sabr* is mentioned in Surah Al-Baqarah (2):156:

- *Who, when disaster strikes them, say, "Indeed we belong to Alláh, and indeed to Him we will return."*

[Al-Baqarah (2):156]

This shows that the consciousness level of those who have *sabr* is in line with the first reality of life that life is a journey from Alláh to Alláh. When individuals have a level of consciousness, they will have peace in their heart because whatever happens in this world is only temporary, and eventually all of us will return to Alláh. The message that everything will return to Alláh is the key reminder to heal anxiety and sadness. This message will instil hope to the heart that will energise the individual to get up and move on.

An ever-growing heart

The seventh indicator of psychological health is an ever-growing heart. In Arabic, this is called tazkiya. So this is the defining indicator of a healthy heart. First of all, human life is not stagnant, but rather it is always dynamic and the experience is always changing. How can an individual become peaceful if what they are facing is always changing and is up and down? Again, a peaceful heart is not a permanent condition, but it is also evolving along with the lifespan. In order to be able to experience peace in the ever-changing environment, the heart should not be fragile, it should not miss anything that creates emptiness, it should be coherent so that it will be sustained, it should be capped in balance, it should be resilient and, finally, it should also be developing overtime. An ever-growing heart is the heart that can expand its understanding and always become broader in knowledge and wiser in understanding. In order to be able to always grow, the heart should always be open for learning.

The meaning of growing in case of tazkiya has a special prerequisite. Before growing, the heart should be purified first so that it will be growing in a purified way. We can say this purification is represented by solidness, fullness, coherence, balance and resilience. The result of this purification and growth of the heart is a peaceful heart. This is to say that the seventh indicator of psychological health is actually connected to each indicator in a systematic way. Within each indicator, there is a strong connection with other indicators in a systematic way.

Mental health is defined by the World Health Organisation (WHO) as consisting of four indicators: (1) cope with daily stressors, (2) realise their abilities, (3) learn well and work well and (4) contribute to their community. If we relate the WHO definition to the definition outlined earlier, then coping with daily stressors is one manifestation of a resilient spirit. And this toughness determines wholeness and balance, as well as harmony of the soul. The second indicator, namely, to realise their abilities, is the initial stage of an ever-growing soul that is always able to understand one's own condition and position for further development. The third indicator, namely, learn well and work well, is also a manifestation of a developing soul that is open so that it can always learn and contribute to its professional life. Likewise, the fourth indicator, namely, contribution to their community, is a manifestation of a developing soul that has the capacity to share with its environment. However, the WHO definition does not yet explain the state or condition of a healthy mind that is ultimately able to overcome problems, learn and contribute. One thing that is not included in the WHO definition is a calm soul, one that is not anxious or worried about the turmoil of life in this world. In fact, mental peace is actually the peak of true mental health.

References

Dawkins, R. (2016). *The God Delusion*. Black Swan.

The Noble Qur'ân Encyclopedia. (n.d.). *English translation – Saheeh International*. https://quranenc.com/en/browse/english_saheeh

4 The seven principles of tazkiya therapy

In this chapter, the concept of tazkiya will be explained in detail including the object, the process and the purpose. This chapter will also explain about the boundaries and the enabling factors of tazkiya therapy and examine tazkiya therapy based on seven principles. These principles serve as guidelines and include the basic assumption, the direction and the rules that tazkiya therapy has to comply with. In this book, what is meant by the "heart" is the spiritual heart, which is the core of the human soul (*nafs*). Since the heart is the core of the soul, both terms are used interchangeably to refer to the essence of the individual.

These principles are (1) knowledge is the best medicine, (2) tazkiya is the process to purify and grow the heart, (3) purification should be started by detachment of the heart from material possessions, (4) respecting privacy is a protective factor of a purified heart, (5) the purpose of tazkiya therapy is to reach happiness in the Hereafter, (6) the process of tazkiya is an interplay between the readiness of the heart and Alláh's guidance and (7) tazkiya therapy is a learning process for both the therapist and the client.

Knowledge is the best medicine

Knowledge in this context is derived from the Qur'ânic term *al-'ilm*. Based on the first five verses of Surah Al-'Alaq (96):1–5, the meaning of *al-'ilm* is the knowledge about the truth based on Alláh's guidance that is written in the Qur'ân and also that is directly given by Alláh to the humankind. According to the Qur'ân, the term *al-'ilm* is a knowledge that is based on *ayat*, which is the sign that is sent down by Alláh through the Qur'ânic verses and the universe to the human souls.

The Qur'ânic verses are the main source of knowledge that can be integrated with the knowledge acquired from natural science and psychosocial science. Therefore, there are three sources of signs or evidence that make the foundation of evidence-based knowledge: the Qur'ânic verses, the natural

DOI: 10.4324/9781032717340-4

phenomena and the dynamics of human souls. The following Qur'ânic verse from Surah Fussilat (41):53 explains this issue:

- *We will show them Our signs in the horizons and within themselves until it becomes clear to them that the Qur'ân is the truth. But is it not sufficient concerning your Lord that He is, over all things, a Witness?*

Based on the Qur'ânic *ayat* above, Qur'ânic verses are the guiding principles of knowledge that can be integrated with the science of nature and the science of human psyche and other social sciences. Therefore, in this book, the three sources of knowledge are integrated to construct a comprehensive understanding about the dynamic of the human psyche (*nafs*) and how to heal its diseases. This principle justifies that tazkiya therapy is a theoretically rich intervention.

Knowledge that is based on *ayat* in the universe, in the human soul and in the Qur'ân functioned as a guidance for human beings in living their lives in this world and also to heal any diseases in the spiritual heart. The Qur'ânic message concerning the relationship between knowledge and healing is mentioned in Surah Yunus ayat 57 as follows:

- *O mankind, there has come to you instruction from your Lord and healing for what is in the chest and guidance and mercy for the believers.*
  [Yūnus (10):57]

This Qur'ânic ayat mentioned that the revelation from Alláh will heal what is inside the chest (*ṣhudur*). When the Qur'ân mentioned "what is in the chest," it means the spiritual heart. This statement means that from the Qur'ânic revelation, which is the *Ilm will heal the heart from its diseases*, the disease of the heart is what we call a psychological problem. Therefore, this ayat justifies that knowledge plays the role as the medicine for psychological problems.

This principle is also adopted by Abu Zaid Al-Balkhi to introduce what is called by Malik Badri as "Cognitive Behavior Therapy of a Ninth Century Physician" (Badri, 2013). Al-Balkhi identified four basic psychological problems that can be cured by knowledge. These four psychological problems are 1) anxiety, 2) depression, 3) anger and 4) obsession. Rania Awaad and Ali (2015, 2016) identified that these four psychological problems are also adopted in the Diagnostic and Statistical Manual of Mental Disorder (DSM-5) with a similar description. These facts justified that knowledge through the intervention of cognitive behavioural therapy can heal the fundamental psychological problems.

The process of healing the spiritual heart from its diseases is called tazkiya. This is mentioned in Surah Ash-Shams verse 9.

- *Successful indeed is the one who purifies their soul.*
  [Ash-Shams (91):09]

Furthermore, the Qur'ân explains that tazkiya needs to be initiated by acquiring proper knowledge. There are three verses in the Qur'ân that explain the connection among knowledge (*al-'ilm*), tazkiya and wisdom (*ḥikmah*). In these verses, knowledge is represented by a revelation that teaches human beings something that they did not know before and corrects them from wrongdoing. These three verses are as follows:

- *Just as We have sent among you a messenger from yourselves reciting to you Our verses and purifying you and teaching you the Book and wisdom and teaching you that which you did not know.* [Al-Baqarah (2):151]
- *Certainly did Alláh confer favour upon the believers when He sent among them a Messenger from themselves, reciting to them His verses and purifying them and teaching them the Book and wisdom, although they had been before in manifest error.* [Āl-'Imrān (3):164]
- *It is He who has sent among the unlettered a Messenger from themselves reciting to them His verses and purifying them and teaching them the Book and wisdom – although they were before in clear error.* [Al-Jumu'ah (62):2]

From the Qur'ânic verses above, there is Alláh as the one who teaches human beings through the revelations, in order to purify our heart, which will result in *ḥikmah* (wisdom). The revelation is the source of knowledge that is used to purify the heart (tazkiya) as the process of healing, and wisdom is the accumulation of knowledge that will heal the spiritual heart from not knowing and wrongdoing. This means that a healthy heart is the one that possesses knowledge and is inspired to do the right thing. This healthy heart is what tazkiya therapy is trying to achieve.

Tazkiya is the process to purify and grow the heart

Tazkiya is an Arabic word that has three meanings. Firstly, it means to purify; secondly, it has the meaning of nourish; and thirdly, it has the meaning of to grow or to elevate. Therefore, tazkiya is a word that represents a process of growing, but the growth should be on the path that is purified. The object of tazkiya is the spiritual heart, which is the core of the human soul.

As the object of tazkiya therapy, the soul is the translation of the Qur'ânic term *al-nafs*, and the heart is a translation of the Qur'ânic word *al-qalb*. The heart is the core of the soul that represents the faculty of the soul that will determine the quality of the individual. This argument is based on the hadith by Rasulullah SAW as follows:

- *In the body there is a piece of flesh, and the whole body is sound if it is sound, but the whole body is corrupt if it is corrupt. It is the heart.*

(Bukhari & Muslim)

In the perspective of tazkiya therapy, the heart consists of the mind, the emotion and the spiritual connection with Alláh. In order to grow the mind, the emotion and the spiritual connection with Alláh, an individual needs to discipline themselves so that the heart is free from diseases. The diseases of the heart will be elaborated in other parts of this book and consists of random desires, selfishness, anger, disorientation, anxiety and so on.

The dynamics of tazkiya therapy as the process of healing the spiritual heart can be referred to in the Qur'ân Surah Al-Hajj ayat 52–54 as follows:

- *Whenever We sent a messenger or a prophet before you O Prophet and he recited Our revelations, Satan would influence people's understanding of his recitation. But eventually Alláh would eliminate Satan's influence. Then Alláh would firmly establish His revelations. And Alláh is All-Knowing, All-Wise.*

[Al-Hajj (22):52]

- *All that so He may make Satan's influence a trial for those hypocrites whose hearts are sick and those disbelievers whose hearts are hardened. Surely the wrongdoers are totally engrossed in opposition.*

[Al-Hajj (22):53]

- *This is also so that those gifted with knowledge would know that this revelation is the truth from your Lord, so they have faith in it, and so their hearts would submit humbly to it. And Alláh surely guides the believers to the Straight Path.*

[Al-Hajj (22):54]

The Qur'ânic verses above explain the dynamics of the human heart and the process of healing. Firstly, Alláh guides human beings through His revelation as the basis of knowledge. The basis of knowledge is to purify the heart. Satan will try to hijack this understanding of the guidance from Alláh to misguide human beings. There are three categories of human beings based on the condition of the heart: the first is those who have disease in the heart, the second is those whose heart is already hardened and the third is those who have a purified heart so that they can acquire the knowledge and become wiser. This message explains that in order to be able to receive guidance from Alláh, we need to purify our heart so that it can grow to become wiser. This is the dynamic illustration of tazkiya therapy in practice.

In this book, the term soul and heart are both used interchangeably. This understanding is also explained by Al-Balkhi (Badri, 2013). This multidimensional concept is common in the Qur'ânic terminologies, different from the conventional psychological terminologies that are partial in nature. For instance, theories that only emphasise the biological aspect of an individual, such as neuropsychology, disregard the existence of the human soul. The concept of psychology from an Islāmic perspective integrates all terms into a system of meaning that is multidimensional and comprehensive.

Tazkiya therapy aims to elevate the soul to a higher level of existence, which is to be at the level of comprehension of the purpose of life itself. The purpose of life is to become an individual that has a deep understanding of the meaning of life and is ready to move happily to the next life. Tazkiya therapy is based on the belief that life in this world is very short and temporary, which will be continued by the more eternal life in the Hereafter. The indicators that tazkiya therapy is already successful are as follows:

a. Detachment of the heart from worldly pleasures so that there will be no more regrets or excessive sadness if someone loses people and possessions that they have loved.
b. They will be easier to forgive and free from revenge because they believe that everything that happened to them is a test of their patience and sincerity.
c. They have very strong hope in any situation and condition because they believe that everything is going to be alright in the end.

These indicators of a healthy heart can be referred to the hadith of Rasulullah that explains the opposite condition of the heart when it has disease.

• *The people will soon summon one another to attack you as people when eating invite others to share their dish. Someone asked: Will that be because of our small numbers at that time? He replied: No, you will be numerous at that time: but you will be scum and rubbish like that carried down by a torrent, and Allāh will take fear of you from the breasts of your enemy and last wahn (enervation) into your hearts. Someone asked: What is wahn (enervation). Messenger of Allāh (ﷺ): He replied: Love of the world and dislike of death.*

(Abu Dawud)

This understanding of dynamics of the heart and the soul needs to be communicated to the psychological scientific society so that Islāmic understanding will not be perceived as something exclusive only to the Muslims. In order to bridge this understanding based on Qur'ânic messages and the Al-Hadith with the conventional psychological knowledge, we can use the psychological term that represents the soul and the heart. One scholar who discusses it in the literature of psychology is John Eccles (1994), who argues that the brain is not the core of human beings. He combined the philosophy of Karl Popper and the quantum physics argument to explain his theory. In his book, *How the Self Controls Its Brain*, John Eccles argues that he believes in the existence of the soul and proves empirically that the human brain is influenced by something that is immaterial. In other words, he explains there is a higher level of consciousness that influences the brain. He believes that this higher level of consciousness is the human soul. In his book, he uses the term self to represent his idea about the soul in order to communicate his idea to the psychological scientific society. In psychological literature, the concept of self is understood to be the core of the individual. However, in conventional literature of psychological science, the concept of self is not clearly defined. The contribution of John Eccles is to define the self as the human soul. This definition is very useful to bridge the Qur'ân-based knowledge with conventional psychology.

Tazkiya therapy is an intervention to heal the disease of the heart; it does not directly solve the problem of the body. However, even those who have a healthy spiritual heart will also experience disparities in physical health and vice versa (Al-Balkhi in Badri, 2013). If the disease is in the body, clients need to seek help from medical experts along with the process of tazkiya therapy. We can say that this is the limitation or the boundary of tazkiya therapy. Even though the physical disease and the disease of the heart are not totally disconnected, the disease of the body needs additional treatments along with the treatment of the heart. For example, some cases of depression might be caused not only by psychological problems but also by an imbalance of the hormones of the body (Al-Balkhi in Badri, 2013). In this case, both tazkiya therapy and medication are needed.

Purification should be started by detachment of the heart from material possessions

There are some conditions that resist individuals in the process of tazkiya or can make individuals' hearts not pure. This condition is based on the Qur'ânic messages that contain the root words of tazkiya. Tazkiya itself has the root word that also means zakat or obligation to share individual wealth or material things with people who are in need. It implies that the fundamental element that can decrease the human soul is excessive love of material possessions. Individuals will have some adversities to reach a pure heart in the process of tazkiya if they still have this kind of excessive love. This explanation has also been stated by Imam Al-Ghazali (1993) in his book, *Ihya 'Ulumuddin*, that explains about some diseases of the heart, such as love of material possessions. Ibnu Qayyim Al-Jawziyya also mentioned issues such as sickness of ignorance, desires, delusion, doubts, anxiety, distress, sadness and anger in his book *The Disease and the Cure* (2020). The Qur'ânic message that covers material possessions is in Qur'ân Chapter 3 verse 14:

- *Beautified for people is the love of that which they desire – of women and sons, heaped-up sums of gold and silver, fine branded horses, and*

> *cattle and tilled land. That is the enjoyment of worldly life, but Alláh
> has with Him the best return [i.e., Paradise].*

[Ál-'Imrán (3):14]

If we learn from the Qur'ânic verses that we collect through the root word " ز
ك و," we will find 56 verses, and the word " ز ك و" is mentioned 59 times, and
32 of those verses are about zakat. Zakat is the obligation to distribute 2.5%
of the wealth if the material possessions reach a certain amount that is called
nisab. This implies that the first fundamental element that can contaminate the
heart is the love of material possessions that exceed a reasonable amount. In
Arabic, this wealth is called *mal*, and the attitude that represents attachment
to this *mal* is called *bakhil* (Al-Humazah (104):2; Al-Balad (90):6; Al-Fajr
(89):20; Al-Layl (92):8). If an individual heart still attaches with this excessive love for material possessions, it would be difficult to move forwards in
the process of tazkiya. The Qur'ânic verse for this issue is as follows:

• *Those who pay zakat . . . Paradise as their own. They will be there
forever.*

[Al-Mu'minūn (23): 4&11]

Respecting privacy is a protective factor of a purified heart

In the process to nourish and to grow themselves, individuals need to be considerate to and respectful of others. There are many explanations of the examples of behaviours that can be practised by individuals to be considerate to and
respectful of others. One of the verses is about the rights and privacy of others.
Alláh the Almighty has taught us to respect others' rights and privacy, even
in the context of entering others' houses. It is in the Al-Qur'ân Chapter 24
verse 27–28.

• *believers! Do not enter any house other than your own until you have
asked for permission and greeted its occupants. This is best for you, so
perhaps you will be mindful. And if you do not find anyone therein, do
not enter them until permission has been given you. And if it is said to
you, "Go back,"[986] then go back; it is purer for you. And Alláh is
Knowing what you do.*

[An-Noor (24):27–28]

Respecting others in the process of nourishing oneself is important
because it involves empathy towards others. In the tazkiya therapy process,
individuals should avoid forcing others to follow their interests and seeing
others as worse than them. Therefore, to nourish and to grow the soul, it is

important to be cautious of stereotyping and envying the difference in others' lives. Instead, human beings need to respect differences and learn from each other as mentioned in the Qur'ân Chapter 49 verses 11–13.

- *you who have believed, let not a people ridicule [another] people; perhaps they may be better than them; nor let women ridicule [other] women; perhaps they may be better than them. And do not insult one another and do not call each other by [offensive] nicknames. Wretched is the name [i.e., mention] of disobedience after [one's] faith. And whoever does not repent – then it is those who are the wrongdoers (11). O you who have believed, avoid much [negative] assumption. Indeed, some assumption is sin. And do not spy or backbite each other. Would one of you like to eat the flesh of his brother when dead? You would detest it. And fear Allâh; indeed, Allâh is Accepting of Repentance and Merciful (12). O humanity! Indeed, We created you from a male and a female, and made you into peoples and tribes so that you may get to know one another. Surely the most noble of you in the sight of Allah is the most righteous among you. Allah is truly All-Knowing, All-Aware (13).*
  [Al-Hujurāt (49):11–13]

Concerning the command to respect others, there are verses in the Qur'ân that specially refer to how we should behave towards Rasulullah.

- *believers! Do not raise your voices above the voice of the Prophet, nor speak loudly to him as you do to one another,1 or your deeds will become void while you are unaware.*
  [Al-Hujurāt (49):2]

The verse mentions about how we should respect others by speaking softly. This attitude will protect us and keep us in a purified state. If we violate this principle, there is a risk that our heart will not be purified anymore, and there will be other consequences that might harm ourselves. Furthermore, this attitude of respect also includes how we behave as a guest. We have to be sensitive that out attitude as a guest may sometimes disturb the host. This attitude is one way to strengthen our empathy. By strengthening our empathy, our heart will be more peaceful.

- *O believers! Do not enter the homes of the Prophet without permission "and if invited" for a meal, do not "come too early and" linger until the meal is ready. But if you are invited, then enter "on time". Once you have eaten, then go on your way, and do not stay for casual talk. Such behaviour is truly annoying to the Prophet, yet he is too shy to ask you to leave. But Allah is never shy of the truth. And when you "believers"*

> *ask his wives for something, ask them from behind a barrier. This is purer for your hearts and theirs. And it is not right for you to annoy the Messenger of Allah, nor ever marry his wives after him. This would certainly be a major offence in the sight of Allah.*
>
> [Al-Ahzab (33):53]

The purpose of tazkiya therapy is to reach happiness in the Hereafter

Tazkiya therapy is not only focused on the happiness in this world but also towards the happiness in the Hereafter that is eternal, as mentioned in Qur'ân Chapter 20 verse 76:

- *Gardens of perpetual residence beneath which rivers flow, wherein they abide eternally. And that is the reward of one who purifies himself.*
  [Tā-ha (20):76]

Another condition that prevents individuals from purifying their heart is lust, different from psychoanalytical approaches that emphasise on human beings' pleasure (pleasure principles) in the form of libido (sexual lust). In tazkiya therapy, pleasure is not denied because it is a human thing; rather, it is delayed in some ways so that individuals do not do anything that could harm themselves or others. This delayed pleasure is done because in tazkiya therapy, pleasure in the Hereafter is more important than the worldly pleasure. This explanation is also in accordance with the concept of delayed gratification from Mischel et al. (1972) and Mischel et al. (1989), which showed that it is a healthy attitude that is beneficial for personality development.

The process of tazkiya is an interplay between the readiness of the heart and Alláh's guidance

The process of tazkiya therapy will involve three parties. First is the client, the second is the therapist and the third is Alláh as the Divine Power and Authority. Tazkiya therapy is not done only by the therapist, but rather it is an interaction among the therapist, the client and Alláh the Almighty. This understanding is very important for several reasons. The client has the potential to learn and that can help the process of tazkiya therapy. The therapist, on the other hand, has the knowledge of the method to do the tazkiya, but he/she does not have the experience that the client has. The knowledge of the therapist can be gained from the Qur'ânic messages, the natural sciences or universe and the dynamic of the individual soul. Third, since the focus of tazkiya is the heart, which is the core of the client's self, it is not possible to be manipulated by the therapist without the client's consent. Even Alláh will not change the condition of the client's heart without their consent. This is mentioned clearly in the Qur'ânic ayat as follows:

- *For each one there are successive angels before and behind, protecting them by Allah's command. Indeed, Allah would never change a people's state until they change their own state. And if it is Allah's Will to torment a people, it can never be averted, nor can they find a protector other than Him.*

  [Ar-Ra'd (13):11]

- *This is how Allah seals the hearts of those unwilling to know the truth.*

  [Ar-Rūm (30): 59]

Adding to that, the clients themselves are only pure or develop their heart with Alláh's permission because Alláh has the power to change people's hearts if the individual has the intention to change. It is in the Qur'ânic verses as follows:

- *Have you not seen those who claim themselves to be pure? Rather, Alláh purifies whom He wills, and injustice is not done to them, [even] as much as a thread [inside a date seed].*

  [An-Nisā'(4):49]

- *O believers! Do not follow the footsteps of Satan. Whoever follows Satan's footsteps, then let them know that he surely bids all to immorality and wickedness. Had it not been for Allah's grace and mercy upon you, none of you would have ever been purified. But Allah purifies whoever He wills. And Allah is All-Hearing, All-Knowing.*

  [An-Noor (24):21]

On the client side, before conducting the tazkiya therapy session, it is very important to be willing to go through the process. Tazkiya therapy cannot be forced towards any individual without their consent. For those who believe in God and the Hereafter, this agreement will involve the willingness to submit to God's will and to open their heart for God's guidance. For those who don't believe in God, at least they will be asked to open their hearts and be willing to have a heart-to-heart conversation honestly and sincerely. The willingness to go through the process of heart-to-heart conversation can be documented in a written consent between the therapist and the client. It is written in Qur'ân Chapter 79 verse 18 that this willingness to go through the process of tazkiya is required, as follows:

- *And say to him, "Would you [be willing to] purify yourself."*

  [An-Nāzi'āt (79):18]

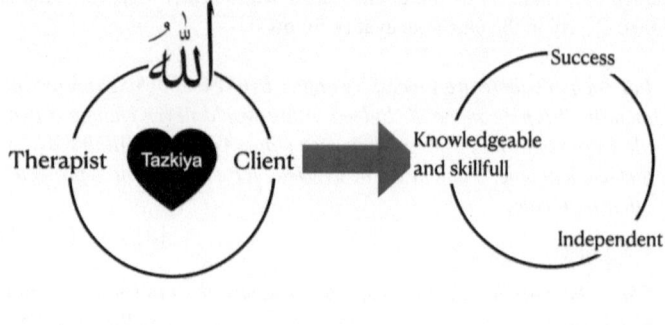

Figure 4.1 Dynamics among the client, therapist and God

Figure 4.1 shows the dynamics of this interaction and the consequences that can emerge from this interaction. These consequences also consist of three dimensions. Firstly, the process of tazkiya therapy will result in the development of knowledge in both the therapist and the client. This shows that the dynamics of tazkiya therapy provides for both the therapist and the client to learn from each other. The second dimension of the consequences is the independence of the client because through the dynamics of tazkiya therapy, the client learns to understand the situation and how to respond to the situation. In other words, through the development of the knowledge and the skills that the client experiences, they will become more independent in dealing with similar psychological problems in the future. If these dynamics happen, then both the client and the therapist will experience success in the interaction, and this success will not be only temporary because it is supported by increasing understanding and independence. Therefore, tazkiya therapy will prevent similar psychological problems from relapsing.

Tazkiya therapy is a learning process for both the therapist and the client

The role of a therapist in tazkiya therapy is to facilitate clients to understand and gain knowledge and skills that can help them purify their soul. In this process, the therapist can optimise the layers of sensing, empathy, reasoning and conscience. The therapist also needs to ask Alláh to purify the clients because the therapist will not know who will be purified. It is important to note in the therapist's mind that his/her role in tazkiya therapy is to help clients, not to heal clients. The therapist should also respect clients because he/she will not know the inside of the client's heart. It is in Qur'ân Chapter 80 verse 3.

- But what would make you perceive, [O Muḥammad], that perhaps he might be purified.

['Abasa (80):3]

Other benefits of this framework of tazkiya therapy are the prevention of feeling proud or guilty from the therapist's side. The success of tazkiya therapy is not because of the therapist's expertise, so the therapist cannot claim it is the result of their competence. The role of the therapist is only a facilitator or a reminder for the client so that the client will understand their situation and what they should do to solve the problem they have. It is Alláh who makes it happen, and Alláh will grant success for the tazkiya therapy if the therapist and the client open their hearts for Alláh's guidance.

On the other hand, when the tazkiya therapy fails, the therapist should not blame themselves for their incompetence because their responsibility is to facilitate the process of tazkiya truthfully and sincerely. Whether the process of tazkiya therapy will be successful or not is not only because of what the therapist did. This way the therapist will be prevented from feeling guilty of failures, and they should always keep the hope for Alláh's help. Feeling proud and feeling guilty are actually also parts of the psychological problem. Therefore, in tazkiya therapy, prayer is also very important. Firstly, the therapist has to pray to Alláh to help them and also ask the client to pray together so that it will open their heart for Alláh's guidance.

Based on the verses above, the therapist in tazkiya therapy helps or facilitates the client to do tazkiya and asks for Alláh's blessings to give the client the opportunity to become better. The therapist does not know which client will end up with tazkiya, so the therapist's job is only to remind and help the client to pray with full hope for Alláh's help. The therapist should not look down on the client because the therapist cannot really know the condition of the client's heart. In other words, the therapist needs to always strive throughout the therapy process. In addition, the therapist also needs to always be patient in interacting with the client and realise that the only one who can purify the therapist and the client is Alláh.

In addition, the therapist needs to have sufficient knowledge about human beings that can be gained through Qur'ânic messages, natural phenomena and the dynamics of the human soul. The dynamics of the human soul itself also can be learnt through psychological and social science. However, findings from the natural sciences and psychological and social sciences need to be in accordance with Qur'ânic messages because Qur'ânic messages provide teachings from Alláh the Most Knowledgeable. Knowledge from Qur'ânic messages and findings in accordance with Qur'ânic messages can help human beings purify themselves in the form of wisdom (*hikmah*). This wisdom can guide human beings to reach their purpose and grow themselves.

Therefore, to become a therapist for tazkiya therapy, one needs to study the Qur'ânic messages, the natural science and psychological and social science

(Fussilat (41):53). This evidence should be coherent with the Qur'ânic messages, meaning that scientific findings that are not coherent with the Qur'ânic messages should be criticised. For example, the current development of neuroscience shows contradicting conclusions. On the one hand, they concluded that human beings have no soul (Harari, 2016; Crick, 1994). On the other hand, Barrett (2017) concluded that the study of the brain revealed that human beings are responsible for their own emotion. Barrett's (2017) conclusion is coherent with the Qur'ânic messages, so her empirical study can be used to enrich the theoretical framework of tazkiya therapy. On the contrary, the conclusion made by Crick (1994) and Harari (2016) are to be criticised by the scientific community so that it is not ready to be integrated for application in tazkiya therapy.

References

Al-Ghazali. (1993). *Revival of religious learning (Ihya' Ulumiddin)*, trans. Fazl Ul Karim (vol. 1). Darul Ishaat.

Awaad, R., & Ali, S. (2015). Obsessional disorders in al-Balkhi' s 9th century treatise: Sustenance of the body and soul. *Journal of Affective Disorders, 180*, 185–189.

Awaad, R., & Ali, S. (2016). A modern conceptualization of phobia in al-Balkhi's 9th century treatise: Sustenance of the body and soul. *Journal of Anxiety Disorders, 37*, 89–93.

Badri, M. (2013). *Abu Zayd al-Balkhi's sustenance of the soul: The cognitive behavior therapy of a ninth century physician*. International Institute of Islāmic Thought; Civilization (ISTAC).

Barrett, L. F. (2017). *How emotions are made: The secret life of the brain*. Houghton Mifflin Harcourt.

Crick, F. (1994). *Astonishing hypothesis: The scientific search for the soul*. Simon and Schuster.

Eccles, J. C. (1994). *How the self controls its brain*. Springer.

Harari, Y. N. (2016). *Homo Deus: A brief history of tomorrow*. Signal Books.

Ibn Qayyim al-Jawziyah. (2020). *The disease and the cure* (trans. O. Hamid). Hikmah Publications.

Mischel, W., Ebbesen, E. B., & Raskoff Zeiss, A. (1972). Cognitive and attentional mechanisms in delay of gratification. *Journal of Personality and Social Psychology, 21*(2), 204–218. https//doi/10.1037/h0032198.

Mischel, W., Shoda, Y., & Rodriguez, M. L. (1989). Delay of gratification in children. *Science, 244*, 933–938.

The Noble Qur'ân Encyclopedia. (n.d.). *English translation – Saheeh International*. https://quranenc.com/en/browse/english_saheeh

5 The protocols of tazkiya therapy

In this chapter, the general protocol of tazkiya therapy will be explained in detail. The protocol of tazkiya therapy consists of three layers. The first thing to do is to ensure that the client is willing to go through the process of therapy. At this moment, the therapist can explain to the client that the tazkiya therapy requires truthfulness and sincerity to explore the psychological problem from a multidimensional perspective. The therapist can also convey to the client that in the process of tazkiya therapy, communication is heart-to-heart interactions. Another thing that the therapist can say to the client is that the therapist wants to learn from any problem that the client has experienced. If the client is religious, it is suggested to start the session with a prayer. By doing that, the client will be aware that there is Alláh who they can rely on.

Another thing that the therapist should keep in mind is to show the four attitudes in order to gain the trust of the client. These attitudes are the system of empathy. The purpose of empathy is to gain trust. In order to gain trust, there are four attitudes that have to be shown and practised during the therapeutic process. These four attitudes are to respect, to care, to be open and to give. To respect is to see the client as an individual who has equal rights and dignity, even though they are currently facing a psychological problem. In other words, never underestimate the client because when the problem is solved, the client might become a wise person. The second attitude is to show care for the client, meaning that the therapist needs to give full attention to the client and show that any problem that the client has is also his/her concern. The third attitude that should be shown to the client is to be open, meaning that the therapist should show the attitude of sharing and active listening, and provide the client with all necessary information, even about personal matters. The fourth attitude that should be shown to the client is the attitude of giving. To show the attitude of giving, sometimes the therapist needs to express that he/she is willing to sacrifice for the sake of the client. If the therapist holds to these principles, relationships based on trust will be obtained, so there will be no more barriers between the client and the therapist. When this happens, any advice or suggestions that are given by the therapist will be accepted by the client. The following is the seven general steps in conducting tazkiya therapy.

DOI: 10.4324/9781032717340-5

These steps are then integrated with the seven approaches that are described below.

- Step 1. The therapist listens empathetically to the client's problems, emotionally and rationally.
- Step 2. The therapist explores further the possible causes of the client's problems by digging into the past experience, emotional dynamics and rational understanding of these experiences.
- Step 3. The therapist leads the client to confirm the core problem that they experienced, which might involve logical fallacy, extreme emotional arousal and a limited perspective of the meaning of life.
- Step 4. If the client is intelligent enough and open minded, they might be able to solve their problem independently after going through step 3. However, the therapist can offer support that can help the client solve their problems.
- Step 5. In order to support the client, the therapist decides where to start by using one of the seven approaches that are available and customises it with the needs of the client.
- Step 6. Once the therapist finds the appropriate approach to the problem of the client, he then goes deeper through the approach to help the client solve the core of the problem.
- Step 7. The therapist directs the client's thoughts, emotions and conscience towards the ideal state based on the selected approach.

Different from the other approaches in psychotherapy, tazkiya therapy is very strong in both the empathetic approach and the directive characteristic. The mastery of the seventh theoretical framework will equip the therapists to show empathy to any conditions that are experienced by the client. The empathy here is based on the deep knowledge of human beings. It is not only a technique of building rapport alone. The empathy that is based on the deep understanding of human beings will be sincere and truthful. On the other hand, the seven theoretical frameworks also provide directions for personality development, all the healing processes and a more stable and higher level of maturity. By doing so, both the client and the therapist who go through tazkiya therapy will experience personal growth. In order to do so, the therapist needs to master the seven approaches of tazkiya therapy. These 7 approaches are detailed below.

Remind the client to keep in mind that Alláh is our destination

The first possible issue that the client is facing is when they feel that they are losing the meaning of life. Usually when the client has this experience, they will always question the purpose of their life. When this happens, the therapist can explore what has happened to the client and how this question developed overtime. The client might tell their stories about disappointment, broken heart, frustration, loneliness or failure in life. The therapist should respond to this story empathetically to get into the heart of the client and try to understand the keywords that have caused these problems. The therapist also needs to understand how the clients perceive life in general, how they define life, what they expect in life and what makes them strongly disappointed in their lives. Furthermore, the therapist can deepen the status of the client's spirituality, especially how they think about life after death. By asking this question, the therapist is reminding the client about life after death so that the client can get out from their worldly problems.

Reach the heart of the client and understand the dynamics of it

The second approach to identify the core problem of the client is to reach the heart. Reaching the heart is to understand the belief system of the client. The therapist puts the effort to understand the real problem of the client and not be satisfied only by the argument or the reason or the explanation because it might be only a part of the rationalisation.

Some basic causes of any psychological problem concern traumatic events in the past or the needs for acceptance or the fundamental expectation. These real issues most of the time are clouded by rationalisation. This real issue can also be detected by whether or not the client's explanation is consistent throughout the counselling session. Sometimes, to cover up the real issue, the client might explain the opposite. In this case, we can use the Freudian theory of ego defence mechanism. The difference between the Freudian approach and tazkiya therapy lies in the basic assumption of human motive. Freudian defence mechanism is only focused on covering up the Id or the sexual libido. In tazkiya therapy, the basic assumption of psychological problems includes unfulfilled needs, dissatisfaction, disappointment, guilt, shame and hidden ambition. Another possible cause of any psychological problem is unexpressed anger.

In order to dig into these core issues, the therapist needs to develop trust in the client. When the relationship is already built on trust, the client will open their heart and will say the truth. To get to this state sometimes takes several sessions. For example, when the client has had a traumatic experience in the past, it will not be easy to open up everything at once. The client will slowly unveil the traumatic experience layer by layer because usually they have a feeling of insecurity. They feel insecure because their feeling of a traumatic event is not at once but involves guilty feelings, anger, shame and some feelings of regret. These traumatic events might also be because of the state besides the bad treatment that the client received from others. Naturally, no one wants to be blamed for something bad that happened to them. But in reality, when something bad happens, usually the individual also has a role in that. And these conflicting situations make them uneasy to say all the truth. Therefore, the therapist should provide a psychologically safe environment to the client so that the client would be willing to open up their true concern. One thing that should not be done by the therapist is to give judgement that makes the client perceive it as blaming them. However, the therapist should slowly make the client realise that making mistakes is okay because nobody is perfect. The most important thing is to forgive themselves and move on with their lives.

This approach can be combined with the other approaches depending on the dynamics of the problem. Also, this approach and other approaches can be derived from the seven realities of life that are already discussed in Chapter 2. For example, the fact that all individuals are vulnerable and are facing uncertainty in life is a very fundamental fact that has to be accepted by the client. The understanding of life as a journey from Alláh to Alláh is also useful to guide the client to change their perspective of their problems. However, the therapist has to be sensitive when this message can be delivered appropriately during the therapeutic process.

Stimulate the client's reasoning, strengthen their empathy and awaken the conscience

The third approach that can be applied in tazkiya therapy is based on the reality that all human beings have four basic potentials, which are sensing, reasoning, empathy and conscience. Psychological problems could happen because of contradiction between these potentials or an imbalance among them. For example, when a couple has a problem, usually the husband says things more rationally, and the wife is more emotional in responding to life issues. Men, especially when their profession is related to technology or accounting, will respond to any life issues with a rational approach. On the other hand, a woman who has multiple roles, whether she is a housewife or a career woman, perceives life problems in a more complex manner. It means that not everything can be rationalised. Sometimes, intuition is more effective than reason. In dealing with a case like this, the therapist could activate the empathy potential of the husband and, at the same time, help the wife to perceive the problem rationally.

To activate the empathy potential, the therapist can challenge the reasoning of the husband who shows that, in reality, relationships can become better when emotion is put forwards. Another way to challenge the reasoning is to ask the client to share their experience when reasoning does not work. Adding to that, the therapist could remind the husband about the purpose of the relationship, which will involve compatibility and understanding that their roles are complementary.

The approach to the wife is to activate reasoning. The therapist can ask the wife to see the issues from a rational perspective. This way, the wife is expected to understand how the husband thinks about issues. Then the therapist can also remind the wife that the differences do not have to become a conflict. Again, differences can complement each other.

Another case that could happen is when the client has what is called the sensing mentality. Sensing mentality is the most severe psychological problem because reasoning, empathy and conscience do not function well. An individual who has a sensing mentality will be driven just by sensation, for example just for fun. When an individual has problems with sensing mentality, they do not have the sensitivity about the purpose of their behaviour or the reason for it. The problem is this individual also does not have a feeling of responsibility, and they do not feel guilty of what they have done. One example of this individual who has a sensing mentality is a bully. A bully will intimidate and press other people just for fun. They do not feel responsible for the consequences of their act of bullying. Actually, the attitude of a bully is because of the emptiness of their heart that might be caused by the relationship with their parents. Their heart does not feel a connection with their parents – this is why they do not develop empathy. Because their empathy is not working, they do not have empathy for their victim. When this bully is under the supervision of the parent, the approach of tazkiya therapy should involve the parent in the family session. The effort that the therapist should do is to reconnect the bully and the parents heart to heart. Achieving that purpose might take several steps – making the parents realise the issue and making the bully understand that what they are doing is not only harmful for the victim, but it will also fire back to himself.

Help clients identify their true meaning in life

The next approach in tazkiya therapy is to focus on identifying the true meaning. It is undeniable that every individual has a certain meaning in their lives. The problem is since human beings have the freedom to develop their own perspective subjectively, their belief about meaning is diverse. Some people might define meaning wrongly if they hold on to false meaning. Those who are holding on to false meaning will experience psychological problems.

A true meaning has certain characteristics that are different from a false meaning. The orientation of true meaning is to contribute, to benefit others and also themselves. On the other hand, a false meaning is only concerned with themselves, or is self-oriented. A true meaning is long-lasting or long-term-oriented, while a false meaning is usually short-term-oriented. An example of false meaning includes ambition to achieve something, revenge or trying to achieve self-oriented satisfaction. An example of true meaning is willingness to contribute for the benefit of everybody, the quest for justice, caring for others and expanding knowledge and wisdom.

The symptoms of those who hold on to false meaning include disappointment, dissatisfaction, feeling of failure and giving up. The approach to heal this psychological problem is to reframe the mindset towards true meaning. The therapist can use the following phrases: "have you ever considered your problem from different perspectives?"; "Can you think about the blessing in disguise of your experience?" and "You know what, actually what you experience is beneficial for you?"

Here is a short case example of this approach. A girl came to a therapist in despair. She told the therapist that her boyfriend has just betrayed her, and it hurts so much. The therapist responds to her by saying "That's good! You know what? You are just safe from a liar. You have to be grateful you found out about this issue earlier, so now you are free to make a new relationship with a good man."

Guide the client to embrace uncertainty and strengthen hope

The fifth approach in tazkiya therapy concerns the reality of uncertainty in life. Concerning the issue of uncertainty, there has been a body of literature that concludes that intolerance of uncertainty is the initial cause of many psychological problems. Intolerance of uncertainty can result in anxiety or depression. This is because someone does not tolerate uncertainty, meaning they reject the reality of life. Since nobody can avoid uncertainty, the only way to face uncertainty is to embrace it. Embracing uncertainty does not mean that we should only go by the flow, but rather that we have to manage ourselves to always adjust to the reality of uncertainty. There are terms that relate to this strategy, for example adaptation, adjustment and agility. Embracing uncertainty is the essence of all those terminologies. The closest psychological modality in adjusting to uncertainty is hope. Hope is defined as a belief that beyond uncertainty there will be something good.

A client who has problems related to intolerance of uncertainty usually shows symptoms of anxiety or frustration or disappointment. The source of these problems is usually expectations that are unfulfilled. Expectation is an attitude that demands certainty. In other words, when an individual has a strong expectation, he/she does not want any surprises. This attitude can be categorised as intolerance of uncertainty. The approach that can be used to solve this problem is converting expectancy into hope. The main difference between expectation and hope lies in the tolerance of uncertainty. When we tolerate uncertainty, we are ready for multiple possibilities that sometimes are unexpected. The power of hope will make these possibilities become opportunities.

Another dimension that relates to uncertainty and hope is risk. When the therapist suggests the client to embrace uncertainty, this also means that they have to be aware and cautious about the risk, which is the possibility of negative results. The dynamics of risk, uncertainty and hope will result in five psychological states. These five psychological states are (1) the psychological state of learned helplessness, (2) the psychological state of optimum challenge, (3) the psychological state of fatalism, (4) the psychological state of optimum opportunity and (5) the psychological state of the comfort zone. Only one of these five psychological states is the healthy psychological state, which is the psychological state of optimum opportunity. The psychological state of learned helplessness will end up in depression. The psychological state of optimum challenge will result in exhaustion or fatigue. The psychological state of fatalism will make the individual idle, only go with the flow and always swinging. The psychological state of the comfort zone will result in the attitude of ignorance and carelessness.

There are four possible issues that are experienced by a client from this approach. A client who has suffered from a psychological state of learned helplessness will show the symptoms of frustration or depression. The direct cause of this symptom is because they are losing hope. They develop the mindset that there is nothing they can do to solve their problem. The problem might come from issues that are already mentioned in the second approach above, that is disappointment, guilt, feeling hurt or the inability to move on from a certain problem. What the therapist should do first is to identify the root cause and from there build hope so that the client will be able to see opportunities to solve that problem. Hope can be narrated in various ways based on the root cause of the problem. Again, this approach is not a distinct approach but can be and should be integrated from other approaches in order to be effective.

The approach of tazkiya therapy to deal with the psychological state of optimum challenge is as follows. Firstly, the client should be reminded that they have a choice to avoid this crisis by creating a habit of early preparation and not waiting until the last minute to finish any task. Secondly, in the process of tazkiya therapy, the therapist can assign an exercise for the client to experience and realise the difference between finishing a test at the last minute and doing the test gradually to prevent critical situations. For example, the client will be assigned to do ten tasks in a week, broken down into seven parts. From day 1 until day 3, the client is assigned to finish one task per day. Then, on days 4 and 5, they should finish two tasks per day. And finally, on days 6 and 7 they should finish three tasks to complete the assignment. After they have done these tasks, the clients are asked their experience to compare it with their habits to do things in the last minute. Then the client is suggested to practise this method to finish any other task in the future.

To deal with the client who has a psychological state of fatalism, sometimes shock therapy is needed. Some cases of fatalism happen in students who do not have motivation to study, are lazy and do not care about their future. These attitudes are the symptoms of fatalism. The cause of this attitude might be previous treatment from their parents who are very strict and always put pressure to study hard. When the pressure is overdone, it will cause resentment. When a client is having the psychological state of fatalism, their awareness of risk and their power of hope are very weak; that is why they are not motivated in any way. To treat this condition, there are two conditions that can be applied: firstly, provoke the awareness of risk, and secondly, develop the power of hope. To design the intervention concerning the risk and hope, first of all the therapist should understand the things that the client considered as meaningful to them. Based on these meaningful issues, the therapist can design the intervention.

The psychological state of a comfort zone will make an individual overly confident. Usually when they are still in that state, they do not think they need help. However, when things go bad, they will be very surprised and cannot accept the reality, and might end up in depression or frustration. One example of this incident can be observed in those people who experience post-power syndrome. People who have post-power syndrome cannot accept any sudden changes in their life, for example a change from a condition where everything is easy to get to a condition that forces them to rely fully on themselves. Sometimes this involves a sudden drop in income and the loss of influence. Intervention for this condition is better performed in a preventive manner. The main message for those who have the psychological state of a comfort zone is that they have to be ready when their condition changes dramatically. In an organisational setting, there are programmes for retirement preparation.

The psychological state of a comfort zone can also happen to students or athletes who are always on the top. Being on the top is actually a very fragile position because the only pathway after the top is the path of going down. Some artists even commit suicide when they cannot accept losing their popularity.

In the approach of tazkiya therapy, which deals with these problems, the first step is to make the client realise their condition and their mindset. Then in the second step, the therapist can make the client explore possibilities beyond their perspectives. This exploration can be in the form of "what if" statements. For example, the therapist can say to the client, "When bad things happen to them, how can they prevent this bad thing from happening?" Another option is to tell the client to imagine opportunities that he/she will miss if he/she does not do anything to grab the opportunity. The problem of the individual with this psychological state is that they don't realise their problem. They don't realise that their attitude causes problems with their surroundings. It is quite a challenge for the therapist to change this perspective.

To deal with the psychological state of a comfort zone, the approach of tazkiya therapy is to make the client reflect on life stories of other peoples and comprehend the uncertainty that always happens in people's life. This is important because usually individuals with the psychological state of a comfort zone are self-oriented, and they think that they are different from other people. They assume that they have special privileges because of their constant achievement in the past.

Guide the client to orient their life towards virtues

The sixth approach of tazkiya therapy is based on the reality that human beings are vulnerable, and they need anchors to hold on. A healthy anchor is a virtue. When an individual is anchored to virtues, they will always find meaning in their life, and they will always have a strong hope about the future. Virtue is a wisdom that is eternal and universal. However, some individuals might orient their anchor to themselves, others or materials. These three alternative anchors are problematic.

When an individual anchors towards themselves, they seem to have self-confidence, but they forget or disregard the need to rely on others. Or sometimes this attitude might not be seen as problematic. They will feel the excitement of being independent and self-reliant. However, their self is not always stable and might fluctuate across time. Another problem is that for some issues, people have to work together to solve problems. Relying on oneself will not be enough. When a problem appears, the individual might develop symptoms of dissatisfaction to themselves and may become guilty and blame themselves for not being strong all time.

Even if individuals orient anchor to others, they might not feel safe and secure if others that they depend on are reliable and dependable. However, other people cannot always be there for them. Others can become weak or even betray. If this condition happened, those people who depend on others might lose hold on their life. They will develop symptoms of confusion, feeling incompetent and feeling lost.

When material is the anchor, such as wealth or properties, an individual will develop an attitude of greed and sometimes anxiety of losing their properties. Usually people who anchor themselves to material things will have a bad attitude towards others and also towards themselves. Their measure of success and happiness is related to material possession. The more they have, the greedier they will be.

Remind the clients to be responsible, hopeful and humble

The seventh approach of the tazkiya therapy is based on the reality that in any life event, all individuals will experience the dynamics of freedom, uncertainty and vulnerability. These three realities in life are undeniable, meaning that psychological problems will occur when an individual denies any of these realities. When a client complains about their inability to make decisions, they deny the principles of freedom. When a client complains about the condition that they do not want, it means that they deny the uncertainty of life. When a client claims to be strong and does not want to accept other people's help, they deny the reality of human vulnerability.

There are three healthy attitudes in every problem, namely, to be responsible, hopeful and humble. These three attitudes have to be expressed simultaneously. A tazkiya therapist should develop sensitivity to these multidimensional attitudes so that they can help the client balance these attitudes. The role of the therapist is to remind the client to always keep in mind these multidimensional attitudes before responding to any problem.

Here are some case examples of these dynamics. A client came to a therapist and complained about her colleague showing some disturbing attitude towards her. This disturbing attitude makes her feel uneasy, and this makes her become unproductive and anxious in her job. She implied that she expected her colleague to stay away from her and not bother her anymore. To deal with this issue, a therapist should enquire to understand the whole story because the client only tells the story from her side. The therapist can ask why the colleague did it to her. Does her colleague only show this attitude towards her? Or does he also treat any woman in the same way? The purpose of this question is to understand whether there is some attitude of the client that caused her colleague to respond. The idea behind this is that everything happens for a reason. What a therapist is trying to do is to remind the client that she is also responsible to some extent of what she has experienced.

This kind of approach has to be done very carefully because the client might feel that the therapist does not want to take her side. And if this happens, the client will not trust the therapist anymore.

The further step of this intervention is to remind the client that she should get help from anybody who is close to her because she cannot deal with this issue by herself. Seeking help is one of the indicators of humility. Being responsible is the expression of independence, but it is not enough because at the same time the client is also vulnerable. That is why, being independent and seeking help at the same time is the best strategy to protect oneself. If we relate this approach to the previous approach, being responsible and at the same time seeking help is the practice for anchoring to virtues. When a client only exercises a responsibility, she is anchoring to self. And when the client depends on others and does not want to be responsible, she is anchoring to others.

When a client is already able to be independent and at the same time seek help from others, what she should do next is to develop hope in her heart. This means that by doing that she should strengthen her belief in the positive

outcome of her effort, even though the result can be in the form of many possibilities. For example, when we relate to the case mentioned above, the result
might be that the colleague who always bothered her will stay away from her
or maybe he will change the attitude because he respects her more, knowing
that the client is acting wisely.

6 Case examples

Case 1: The case of Nurul (losing meaning)

Nurul (pseudonym) is a new student of the biggest university in the country. Being a new student in this university is actually something to be proud of, and most people will be very happy. However, Nurul reports that she feels uneasy lately, and she spends most of her time staying at her dormitory room by herself. At the counselling session, she told me about the story of her life. Her parents were divorced when she was still a little girl. They put her in her grandma's house, and she has been living there until now, raised by her loving grandma. Actually, Nurul was a happy teenager, and she didn't feel that her parents' divorce was a big problem because she can still meet them periodically but not at the same time. Nurul grew up well, and her appearance shows that she is a good Muslim. She dressed up in humble clothing and wore a hijab. Initially, she was talking about Islāmic psychology and showed interest in studying it more. The way she talks is polite and humble, and she shows sincerity in her curiosity.

Her grandma lives around 365 km away from the city where she studies right now. Therefore, she had to move and live by herself in the dormitory. She reports that her friends in her department and also in the dormitory usually go home on holidays or weekends. They go to their parents, and they express cheerfulness when it happens. Nurul felt that she didn't have a home to go on holidays, and she started to feel that she is different from her friends because she doesn't have a father or mother to go home to. Recently, she realised that grandma's house is not quite a home for her and makes her feel incomplete. This feeling grows day by day, and it is getting worse. She started to question the meaning of life. She started to feel that she is not having a normal life and felt lonely every time she reflected about this condition. When I asked her, "What was the most disturbing feeling that she is experiencing right now?" She answered that she doesn't understand the purpose of her life anymore. She cannot join her friends when they are having fun, and she doesn't feel like going out with her friends anymore. She feels that her life has no meaning.

DOI: 10.4324/9781032717340-6

Nurul's condition is currently not quite severe. However, if she keeps thinking and feeling this way, she could experience depression that is prone to suicidal tendency. Understanding this condition and considering that she is actually a practicing Muslim, I then responded to Nurul's confusion by saying, *All human beings will eventually go home and go back to Alláh 📿. So, the purpose of your life in this world is to prepare yourself, so that you will be ready when you go home to Alláh 📿. That is the most important thing that you should keep in mind. And the problems that you face in your life are not significant as long as you remember that the most important thing for you to do is to keep doing good deeds and useful things so that you will be ready when you meet Alláh 📿.*

Hearing this statement, Nurul seemed to realise that this is something that actually she had already known before but recently was clouded by her sadness and confusion. She looked relieved and showed that she understood this reality. She expressed that she is thankful for this session. She went home and felt relieved as if she was free from a heavy burden.

Case analysis

In this case, Nurul is an example of those who already have belief in Alláh but this belief in Alláh was hijacked by her emotion after realising that she is different from her friends in terms of her family condition. Therefore, the therapeutic approach is to remind her and bring her back to the essence of life based on the Islāmic belief system. This approach cannot be applied to clients who do not have this state of spiritual belief. If we apply this approach to those who are not ready, then it will be classified as spiritual bypassing.

The case of Nurul illustrates the brief method of tazkiya therapy. It seems that it is very simple and short, but it reflects a psychological dynamic that can be explained by a number of theories. What I did to Nurul is not merely changing her behaviour or her thoughts, but it touches her heart. I picked the word "home" as the keyword as it serves as the window to Nurul's heart. Therefore, I focus on the word "home" that Nurul is longing for, to touch her heart and build on it the essential meaning of "home" for the soul. The true and real home of the soul is heaven, where we will meet Alláh.

Case 2: The case of Ana (bipolar disorder)

Ana is a 30-year-old woman. She is the first child of four siblings. Her father died when she was in middle school. She lives with her mom, her younger brother and two younger sisters. Her mother is a very simple housemother who does not have a stable income, but they're supported by their big family for their daily needs. Since several years ago, Ana has been showing unstable emotion and has been hostile to her mother and her siblings. She always seeks attention, especially from her mother, and she will be very angry when what she wants cannot be fulfilled by her mother. However, when everything is okay, she can become a sweet girl, especially when she meets her big family. She was diagnosed with bipolar disorder. Her big family, the siblings of her mother, became concerned with her condition because her mother is very often consulted and asks for help from the big family to handle her.

Her father was very dominant in her family. Even though her family's socio-economic status was not quite strong, her father was very confident and very active in the neighbourhood. He was active in social organisations and had a strong influence on the neighbours. The neighbours respected him because he has a very wide social network. He didn't have a stable job, but he always found things to do, like buying and selling goats and he once opened a simple eating place. He was also active in a political party and was once elected as a member of the local house of representatives. He was very confident, and he sometimes treated Ana's mother and also all his children roughly.

Ana's mother has a simple personality. She also has low self-esteem and always treats her children to be "humble," meaning she taught her children that they do not deserve to do or to play with the relatives from the big family. For example, when her relatives were playing a computer game and Ana showed interest and wanted to try, her mother said, "You cannot do that. That is not for you." Her mother always sees her family as a lower class that does not deserve the privilege of the big family, who are more educated and also more wealthy.

Ana grew up with low self-confidence, and she has been having problems with schooling. She went to the local school that has low quality, and she mingled with kids from the neighbourhood who are uneducated. Once when she was younger, she had a relationship with a boy who was in a gang. Knowing about the relationship, the big family was concerned, so the uncle and the aunt tried to advise her not to continue the relationship. It seems that she was disappointed with this incident. She felt the pressure from the big family and tried to rebel. One expression of her rebellious behaviour is that she often quits from something that she has started. For example, once she was sent to a training programme that was scheduled for 7 days, but she quit on the second day without any clear reason. In another incident, when she was given the opportunity for a job, she also quit after a few weeks.

Entering the age of 30, Ana became a trouble for her family. She was so bossy to her younger brother and sisters that it made them kind of afraid of her. She always wants to control everyone in her family to serve her needs. Her brother and sisters became intimidated and insecure living with her. Her mother felt powerless and didn't know what to do and was even almost frustrated with this condition. Knowing this, her aunts suggest her brother and sisters to move out from the home and stay with the family's house, but this idea made Ana very angry and to intimidate her siblings even more. The condition of her family became a common concern of the big family, and one of her aunts suggested Ana to see a psychologist.

The psychologist diagnosed Ana as having a borderline personality. From the counselling sessions, it was found that Ana was actually anxious and wanted to get married and hasn't got anyone to marry. Actually, her younger brother already has somebody that he wanted to marry, but Ana doesn't let her brother get married before her. The therapist tried to make Ana understand that marriage is one of the life events that is not fully in our control. The therapist said further that marriage can only happen when Alláh permits it to happen. The therapist suggested Ana to pray to Alláh and be more patient. Several sessions are needed to convince Ana about this perspective. Actually, Ana is also a practising Muslim, and for her, praying to Alláh is not something new. However, currently she does prayer as part of the religious ritual only.

A few months later, the therapist got the good news that Ana is getting married soon. It happened so fast, and everybody was surprised. Just a week earlier, a relative of his late father came to her house with a man who was also looking for someone to marry. When Ana was introduced to him, they both felt that they are a good fit for each other, and without any delay, the family decided to arrange a wedding for them. The wedding was planned a month later, and everybody was happy. After getting married, Ana's emotions became quite stable, although sometimes she still shows her dominance towards her mother and her siblings. But, after her marriage, Ana is not intimidating anymore although her character is still the same. Her marriage opened the door to her younger brother who also got married, followed on later by her younger sister.

Case analysis

Ana experienced several issues through her lifetime. When she was a little girl, she experienced the dominance of her father and the weak position of her mother. This experience developed a certain mindset for Ana. She was also experiencing a broken heart and felt pressured by the big family. These experiences formed an attitude of revenge in Ana's personality. Revenge is a response to an unhappy experience in the past and also disappointment. One form of revenge is to imitate the person who gave her hard times. In this case, she imitates her late father.

Ana grew up from an unconfident girl to become the dominant person in the family. This is a form of revenge to her father who was also dominant and rough. Her personality grew along with her age. The older she became, the more anxiety she had. This anxiety grew from unfulfilled expectations. She expected her mother and her siblings to understand her and her condition, but she expressed this roughly like her father. On the other hand, she was very dependent on her mother and her siblings and demanded them to always be around her. This is one of the expressions of those who rely on others as their anchor.

Actually, she needs her family, but at the same time, she was also disappointed with them because they cannot provide what she really wants. This conflicting emotion puts her psychological health in trouble. This is one example of cases with an incoherent heart. Because of the incoherences in her heart, she experienced difficulty finding peace in her heart. This condition made it difficult for her to show empathy to other people.

When she met the therapist, she experienced at least a couple of new perspectives in seeing her life. What the therapist did can be categorised into three steps. Firstly, the therapist showed empathy so that Ana finally could open up about what she really wanted. Secondly, the therapist helped Ana reorient her anchor from anchoring towards others to anchoring towards Alláh. By suggesting this, the therapist actually introduced one of the virtues in life. At the same time, the therapist actually switched Ana's expectation to hope, which is healthier than expectation. When you rely on Alláh, you will slowly grow hope in your heart. This hope is a very strong psychological state that can help Ana get away from anxiety and frustration. Last but not least, the surprising solution that came to Ana is not something that was not arranged by anyone. In tazkiya therapy, this is the evidence of Alláh's intervention to purify and to grow Ana's heart to be more mature.

Case 3: The case of Elena (demotivation)

Elena is a graduate student in educational psychology. Currently she has almost finished the programme and has been working on her final thesis. She came to me to consult about her difficulties in finishing her thesis. She said that she was kind of anxious and found it difficult to concentrate. She is already in the third year of the programme, and the length of the programme should be 2.5 years. Therefore, she is already too late, and this condition adds to her anxiety. This condition made her more anxious and more difficult to concentrate on finishing the thesis.

Before Elena joined the graduate programme, she worked in a private company and earned well. Elena is the only child in her family, and her parents depend on her economically. Elena decided to join the master programme because she said that to be an educator is her true passion. When she worked in a company, she did not feel the satisfaction of what she was doing, and she thought that what she did was not fulfilling her passion. The problem is when she quit the company, which gave her a high income, her parents and her big family were disappointed. She was expected to take care of her parents who are already in their senior ages and did not have a stable income. This expectation causes her quite a pressure that makes her study not enjoyable.

When she was still attending classes, this pressure did not seriously disturb her because what she had to do was just attend the class, study the materials and take the exam. However, when she works on her thesis, there is no more structure, and she has to manage herself on how to make the proposal, how to do the research and so on. At this stage, this pressure really disturbed her, it made it difficult to concentrate and she could not progress on her thesis. Meanwhile, as time passed by and as she is approaching the deadline, if she does not meet the deadline, she is going to be expelled from the programme. That is why, at this time she was in a critical situation and did not know how to solve this issue.

Understanding her situation, I said to her that there are things in life that she cannot control. However, there are some issues that are in her hands, meaning that she has something that she can do, whatever other people say to her. I asked her to identify things that she cannot control and things she can control. I also said to her that whatever will happen in the future is uncertain, but if she can focus on things that she can do, she will have a stronger hope of getting the best result even though it might not satisfy others. I also made her understand that if she did not finish the thesis, things would get worse. She will become a total loser because she already quit her job, and she will not get a degree from the programme. Therefore, the only choice that will give her more opportunity to gain something out of this is finishing the thesis and ignoring the negative comments from her big family, the pressure and also the blame that she received because she had quit a good job to do the master programme.

A few months later, I heard good news that Elena finally finished her thesis and graduated as a master of educational psychology. I did not have the chance to meet her after that, but at least she could move forward with more confidence. She might still have an issue in terms of income, and she might have to face the disappointment of her big family, but that is another issue that hopefully she can deal with because she has already developed new perspectives on facing problems that always have uncertainties attached to them.

Case analysis

Elena's case is an example of tazkiya therapy that does not directly involve the issue of believing in God, meaning this case could happen to anyone, even though they do not believe in God. However, the approach used in the case of Elena is one of the second approaches that is derived from the primary premise about life which involves tolerance to uncertainties, reliance on hope and risk awareness. This framework actually also develops from the reality that life is a temporary journey from Alláh to Alláh. That is why along the way in our life, we should be aware that we are not totally in control and that if we believe in Alláh, we will not lose hope for the solution of any problems.

7 Summary

This book is about tazkiya therapy, a unique approach in psychotherapy from the Islāmic perspective. The main source for tazkiya therapy is Qur'ânic messages and the hadith of the prophet Muhammad SAW. The main unique feature of tazkiya therapy is that it involves Alláh in the therapeutic process. This is very fundamental because it is mentioned twice in the Al-Qur'ân that Alláh is the only one who can make the process of tazkiya happen.

Tazkiya is an active verb meaning to purify and grow the soul. When an individual always does tazkiya, they will gradually develop to be a wiser person. Therefore, tazkiya therapy is not fixing problems, but it is more developing in nature.

In Chapter 2, this book explores the seven realities of life as the basis for diagnosis and therapy to multiple issues in psychological health. These seven realities are (1) life is a journey from Alláh to Alláh, (2) the heart is the core of human self, (3) there are four basic potentials of the human heart, (4) human beings are motivated by meaning, (5) life is a test in the form of uncertainties, (6) human beings are vulnerable and (7) freedom, uncertainty and vulnerability always coexist in every moment of human life.

In Chapter 3, this book describes the seven indicators of psychological health based on the Qur'ânic messages. This book uses the term psychological health to replace the term mental health because the focus of tazkiya therapy is the psyche or the soul, not only the mind. Since the focus of tazkiya therapy is the soul, the perspective of tazkiya therapy is not limited to life in this world, but it reaches out to life in the Hereafter. That is why the ultimate indicator of psychological health is a peaceful heart that will guarantee to enter Heaven as the ultimate happiness. In total, including a peaceful heart, there are seven indicators of psychological health. The seven indicators of psychological health are (1) a peaceful heart, (2) a solid heart, (3) a full heart, (4) a coherent heart, (5) a balanced heart, (6) a resilient heart and (7) an ever-growing heart.

The seven principles of tazkiya therapy are explained in Chapter 4 as the guidance for the practice of tazkiya therapy. These seven principles provide guidance and boundaries of the practice of tazkiya therapy that have to be kept in mind by the tazkiya therapist. These principles are (1) knowledge is

DOI: 10.4324/9781032717340-7

the best medicine, (2) tazkiya is the process to purify and grow the heart, (3) purification should be started by detachment of the heart from material possessions, (4) respecting privacy is a protective factor of a purified heart, (5) the purpose of tazkiya therapy is to reach happiness in the Hereafter, (6) the process of tazkiya is an interplay between the readiness of the heart and Alláh's guidance and (7) tazkiya therapy is a learning process for both the therapist and the client.

Based on the realities of life and the concept of psychological health, Chapter 5 describes the protocol of tazkiya therapy that consists of seven approaches. These seven approaches are not seven different approaches, but a seven-in-one approach. It means that each approach is connected and blended with other approaches. These seven approaches serve as the entry point to psychological problems, but once the problem is identified, the seven approaches can together be used simultaneously and systematically to help the client heal themselves.

In Chapter 6, three real-life case reports are presented to illustrate tazkiya therapy in practice. From these three case reports, the reader can learn how the seven realities of life and the seven approaches of tazkiya therapy set a framework to diagnose and treat the client. One thing that can also be learnt from these cases is that the seven approaches of tazkiya therapy do not have to be applied one by one. The reader can see that in practice, even only one approach can solve a problem as long as the approach is coherent with the diagnosis result.

Tazkiya is an ongoing process as long as the individual lives. It is a process of ever growing, but it is also natural if the individual experiences ups and downs during the process of tazkiya. So, tazkiya therapy is not a one-shot intervention; rather, it is like opening the door for the journey in elevating oneself. It is expected that through tazkiya therapy, the client will become independent and capable of developing their knowledge and elevating their soul to become a wiser person and closer to Alláh. For a professional therapist, the condition of the heart can be seen and felt through the narrative that is expressed by the client and also by the appearance of body language that is shown.

This book is the initial publication of tazkiya therapy that serves as an introduction to the approach. InsyaAlláh when tazkiya therapy becomes common practice, there will be more cases that can be published.

Index